CORE
PERFORMANCE
ESSENTIALS

MARK VERSTEGEN

AND PETE WILLIAMS

CORE
PERFORMANCE
ESSENTIALS

THE REVOLUTIONARY NUTRITION AND EXERCISE PLAN

RODALE

This edition first published in the UK in 2006 by
Rodale International Ltd
7–10 Chandos Street
London W1G 9AD
www.rodalebooks.co.uk

Printed and bound in the UK by CPI Bath using acid-free paper from sustainable sources.

1 3 5 7 9 8 6 4 2

A CIP record for this book is available from the British Library

ISBN-13: 978-1-4050-8813-8
ISBN-10: 1-4050-8813-3

This paperback edition distributed to the book trade by Pan Macmillan Ltd

Notice
This book is intended as a reference volume only, not as a medical manual. The information given here is designed to help you make informed decisions about your child's health. It is not intended as a substitute for any treatment that they may have been prescribed by their doctor. If you suspect that they have a medical problem, we urge you to seek competent medical help.

Mention of specific companies, organizations or authorities in this book does not imply endorsement by the publisher, nor does mention of specific companies, organizations or authorities in the book imply that they endorse the book.

Addresses, websites and telephone numbers given in this book were accurate at the time the book went to press.

RODALE
LIVE YOUR WHOLE LIFE™

We inspire and enable people to improve their lives and the world around them

CONTENTS

v

THE GAME OF LIFE

thlete *n.* A person possessing the natural or acquired traits, such as strength, agility and endurance, that are necessary for physical exercise or sport, especially those performed in competitive contexts.

Everyone is an athlete. Even if you don't play sport, you compete each day in the Game of Life. In order to succeed, you need a strategy to build and maintain the necessary strength and energy to accomplish your goals.

The day-to-day life of a corporate worker, student or stay-at-home parent is just as physically and mentally gruelling as anything you'll find in sport. I work with professional athletes who accomplish tremendous feats, but even the challenges they face sometimes pale in comparison with those that the vast majority of people face every day.

After all, athletes spend most of their time practising for short periods of competition, and they have the benefit of off-seasons. Most of us have no time to practise; the game is going on all the time. There is no off-season, except the occasional holiday. The competition never comes to an end.

Not only that, but we risk a lot more than not making the play-offs or taking home the title. Our performance affects the quality of life and destinies of those we care about most. The stakes could not be higher.

Look at the definition of *athlete* above.

Even if you have never picked up a ball and have no intention of doing so in the future, you need strength, endurance and agility just to get through your daily routines; resist fatigue, frustration and distraction; and meet the demands of life.

For all the talk of creating washboard abs, counting carbs and losing weight, many of us have lost sight of what really matters: improving our physical and mental wellbeing to ensure a productive day-to-day existence, to say nothing of a long and healthy life.

Don't get me wrong; it's important to look great. But why not take the same amount of time and effort that many people invest only in looking good and follow a programme that produces not only cosmetic changes but also increases energy, sharpens your mental edge and reduces and prevents nagging pains in your back, knees and hips?

Sound good to you? Here's some even better news: you don't have to spend hours in the gym, deprive yourself of tasty food or acquire an advanced degree in exercise science to understand this regime.

Core Performance Essentials, as the name suggests, includes everything you need and nothing you don't. The entire programme can be done either at the gym or in the comfort of your own home, with only a minimal investment in equipment. Even then, if you don't want to swallow that cost, there are exercise variations that don't need equipment.

You won't be forced to follow a diet programme that's aggravatingly complicated, impossible to adhere to or ineffective. Instead, you'll learn simple principles and recipes that will trim your waistline and food bills while improving your performance.

Firstly, you need to understand that this is a long-term strategy. You'll notice there's no time-stamped subtitle to this book: no '12 Weeks to a Better You'; no '6-Week Plan for Great Abs'. This is not a quick fix programme, a New Year's resolution or an extreme makeover. I don't want this to be the latest in a series of programmes you try, only to give up when you become bored after a few weeks, get too busy or become frustrated.

After all, even the most successful athletes or businesspeople don't quit after one good or bad season. I've been fortunate to help some of the world's greatest athletes build successful careers, and I want to provide you with similar tools so that you can lead a life of sustained performance and improved long-term health.

Will it take some effort? Of course it will. You must want to bring out the athlete that's inside you. But before you start thinking that this process isn't for you, pay heed to the first rule of investing: *past performance is not indicative of future return.* No matter how badly off you are right now, you're not doomed to poor health and an early exit if you take action now. On the other hand, if you *don't* take action, that past performance – or lack thereof – *will* probably result in an unhappy future return.

Unfortunately, it's an uphill battle. It's easy to be beaten down by this fast-paced culture; it's easy to think you can eat whatever and whenever you want; it's easy to abandon consistent exercise – or abstain from it altogether – and still feel as if you'll come out ahead. So you grind harder, firm in the belief that you can outwork and outhustle anyone through sheer willpower.

Sooner or later, your body will break down due to injury or illness. It's a vicious downward spiral – the harder you work, the more run-down you become and the less energy you have. Nobody can keep up the pace forever unless they have, like the best athletes, a game plan to help them. The idea is to sustain this winning energy level throughout your life.

For instance, let's say you're a successful executive. You wake up in the morning after a short, restless sleep. You rush out of the door and grab a muffin and an expensive, calorie-laden designer coffee on the way to work. While answering e-mail and putting out a few office brush fires, you guzzle fizzy drinks or more coffee. By lunchtime, you're starving, so you grab some a takeaway or head to a restaurant for a meal that offers little nutritional value. By mid-afternoon you're dragging, so you drink more caffeine and get a jolt of sugar from the vending machine. Still, you struggle to get as much work done as you'd like, so you either stay late or take work home, where you eat the first thing you can find, perhaps pizza or pasta. By now, the day is over and your back, as usual, is killing you. You've had no time to exercise. Instead of releasing endorphins and recharging with a workout, you unwind with a few beers or glasses of wine. You're too exhausted to give quality time to your partner or children. It's all you can do to slump in front of the TV for a few hours, snacking on more junk food before collapsing into bed for another short, restless sleep before repeating the process the next day.

Sound familiar?

If not, let's say you're a stay-at-home parent. You're jolted from a brief slumber by a screaming baby, and you stagger around for an hour, dealing with the toddler and getting an older child or two off to school. The youngest commands your attention for most of the day, a whirlwind of nappies, feedings and time with other children. Soon it's the middle of the afternoon and it's time to chauffeur the children to sport, music practices and other extracurricular activities.

Along the way, you must handle the crush

▶

of household routines, the inevitable home maintenance crisis and, oh yeah, the small matter of feeding yourself. Dinnertime arrives and all you've consumed is coffee and a fast-food lunch on the way back from the supermarket. You'd like to work off the extra kilos you've packed on in recent years, but who has the time?

Perhaps you're a student. You wake up too late to have a substantial breakfast, if any, and because you're not allowed to eat in class, you're famished most of the morning. Because of tight budgets, the cafeteria offers little beyond highly processed, high-starch meals, but fizzy drinks and sugary snacks are usually also available. That burst of sugar carries you through part of the afternoon, but soon, you're struggling to stay awake in class and you're even feeling hungry again.

Even though you're tired, you also feel on edge, as if you need to run around, but you don't have time between lecturers. When you finally get home, you're so hungry that you grab the first thing available, which usually is junk food. Course work, phone calls, friends and e-mail take up the afternoon and much of the evening, which includes pizza or a takeaway dinner that your parents or flat-mates brought home.

Remarkably, most people manage to function adequately enough in this fast-forward, time-pressed world to slog through life. But instead of reaching their maximum potential and reaching their goals, they're more like *goalkeepers,* deflecting the shots that life fires at them.

The consequences of this defensive lifestyle are devastating. By eating poorly and not exercising, you're not as productive and you accomplish less. You make poor use of your time at work or school, which takes away from the time you can spend with loved ones, to say nothing of your earning potential. Even when you do have time, you're too tired and stressed to offer love and support to the people who matter most.

Still, you manage to achieve a degree of success at work or college and even find some time to spend with your loved ones. But you feel like the mythical Greek, Sisyphus, doomed to endlessly push a rock up a hill, never getting over the top. A little voice in the back of your head, or perhaps a real voice in the form of a doctor or loved one, keeps reminding you to pay attention to your health and get your life in order, but you never seem to have time.

Bottom line: you need to stop playing goalie. After all, even the best goakeepers can't fend off every shot. But this isn't a game: once your health slips, you're on a downward spiral. And then it's *game over.*

Of course, you're not alone. According to the World Health Organization, 36 million people die each year from causes related to poor diet, physical inactivity and tobacco. Smoking currently kills about 5 million adults a year. That means the rest of those deaths are directly related to diet and physical inactivity.

And it's only getting worse. In the United States, although the death toll from most preventable causes decreased in the decade between 1990 and 2000, deaths caused by obesity and inactivity went up by a mind-boggling 33 per cent. In the majority of European countries there has been a 10–40 per cent increase in obesity in the last 10 years. In Australia the prevalence of obesity has more than doubled in the last 20 years. Similar findings have been reported from developing countries. This increase in obesity has left many countries' health systems struggling to cope with the rise in related health problems.

If healthcare systems are feeling the strain now, what will it be like if things don't change? Obesity already costs the UK economy £2 billion a year according the National Audit Office. Some companies are considering cutting back on health benefits. Obesity is increasingly seen as an insurance risk and life insurance premiums may start to reflect this. Some insurers are already taking applicants' weight into account when offering them health and life insurance.

Still, for some people, the prospect of an early death is not enough to change an unhealthy lifestyle. So let's consider a few more horrors: inactive people are far more likely to suffer from depression and agonizing back problems; they lose mobility earlier in life and no longer can play sport, lift children or even walk; and they're more likely to develop diabetes, which can lead to blindness, kidney failure and loss of limbs. Worst of all, these ailments are kicking in far earlier than in previous generations.

Current healthcare systems worldwide are based on treating the effects of inactivity and poor diet rather than addressing the causes. Money is spent on responding to acute problems, testing, diagnosing, relieving symptoms and seeking a cure. Much less money and effort is spent on preventive health care.

The terrible irony in this crisis is that we soon could see the average life expectancy *decrease,* even though medical technology continues to advance, and even though we know far more about the impact of poor diet and inactivity than ever before.

It's not an exaggeration to say that if this continues, health care systems will collapse and millions will face early death. Everyone will feel the impact.

The stakes are high and, unfortunately, the teams are unfairly matched. In one corner, we have overloaded, overworked, overstressed people, struggling to balance the demands of work and family. They find it difficult to exercise, plan and prepare healthy meals, and take a proactive approach to life.

In the other corner stands a powerful opponent: Western consumerism. Its roster includes wealthy fast-food marketers bombarding us with pitches for their unhealthy, seductively convenient foods, many made with unnatural, high-fat substances.

The opponent's roster has other strong players, including vast cable television universes, the Internet and video games looking to grab our attention. There are cash-strapped school boards forced to sell playing fields and, in some countries, raising money by allowing vending machines and fast-food sponsorship of school lunches. This is great for the companies involved as it means they get people into the habit of eating junk when they're young and impressionable.

It's time to level the playing field – and I'm here to help. For the last 15 years, I've had great success working with athletes at all levels, from those who have won Super Bowl, World Series and World Cup championships to the thousands of people who read my first book, *Core Performance.*

If you missed that book, that's okay. In fact, look at *Core Performance Essentials* as both a prequel and a sequel to *Core Performance.* If you're one of those people facing the challenges discussed above, this is the perfect starting point. This book is designed for time-pressed adults for whom *Core Performance* might be a little too taxing. It's for teenagers who want to get off the couch and establish some good habits at a young age. It's for the person who has never engaged in much physical activity, but who is looking for an effective, easy-to-understand place to start. It's even for the person who wants to augment an existing programme or freshen up a routine that's grown stale.

It's also a sequel for *Core Performance* readers who, for whatever reason, no longer have as much time to commit to a more extensive regime. This is an abbreviated programme that provides the most benefit in the least amount of time.

But this is much more than just another diet and nutrition programme. Too many books give you those components, figuring you'll find a way to make it work. Together, we're going to create a new lifestyle based around your existing commitments and provide you with the motivation and tools to make your better habits permanent.

After all, you have commitments etched in stone in the form of family and work. So you have to establish this athletic mindset and be ready to go, because this isn't just a tennis match or round of golf. The consequences of falling short in life are so much greater than they are in sport.

In short, this book is for you, the competitive athlete in the Game of Life. Here you'll find everything you need – the Core

Essentials – to create a positive lifestyle based on core values, physical activity and healthy eating that will fuel you towards success in every aspect of your life. Your goal is *to live longer and live better.* It's to weave this system into a healthy lifestyle that will be at the heart of everything you do.

Consider *Core Performance Essentials* your new playbook. It's your life – are you ready to get in the game?

MINDSET

NUTRITION

MOVEMENT

RECOVERY

PART

1

THE
CORE
MINDSET

WHAT'S AT YOUR CORE?

S o, now you're thinking we're going to launch into a nutrition and workout discussion? Not so fast. Before we do that, we need to tweak your lifestyle and thought process. If you start a diet and exercise programme without a big-picture lifestyle master plan, you're doomed to fail.

The idea behind this programme is that everything starts from the core. We want to build our lives from the inside out, not just at the superficial level of physical appearance, like so many other programmes.

Core is a popular buzzword. Most people think it refers only to your abdominals, and countless books and articles have been written on how to produce six-pack abs.

But your core, from a strictly physical standpoint, is more than just your abs. As we'll discuss later in the book, the core refers to the mid-section of the body – from hips to shoulders – and is the basis for all movement.

If you look at this as just another diet and exercise programme, you will have a difficult time producing long-term change. That's why I want you to think broader than just nutrition and fitness. Think of this as an integrated lifestyle system with four components, the four parts of what I call the Core Essentials: Mindset, Nutrition, Movement and Recovery.

This diagram was developed in collaboration with our partners at Tignum, the world's leading institute for executive excellence.

When embarking on a new programme of nutrition and exercise, you will be far more motivated if you take a step back and define what drives you. So, don't look at our Core Essentials sphere above as an abstract concept. Instead, think of it as a Super Ball. When I was little, I'd take one of those tiny red extra-bouncy Super Balls and slam it as hard as I could on the driveway. It seemed to go 15 metres in the air, bounce, and then go another 6 metres. I marvelled at the power of this simple object smaller than a golf ball. Indeed, the reason a golf ball can travel so far is that there's the equivalent of a Super Ball at its core.

We want to create a Super Ball in your own core, not just through nutrition and exercise but by rewiring your mindset and incorporating recovery into your lifestyle. Let's take a brief look at each of these four components.

MINDSET

The simple fact that you picked up this book suggests that you have, to some degree, the proper mindset you'll need to make the necessary changes in your life.

I once had the wonderful opportunity to chat with John Wooden, perhaps the greatest college basketball coach of all time. He told me that he always looked for players who were not just willing, but *eager,* to do what it takes. Until a player was eager to become the best he could be, Wooden said, there was no use in him showing up for practice.

On the surface, that might seem like a minor distinction. But think of the relationship that most people have with their jobs. They're willing to show up for work – after all, they presumably need the money – but not really eager to do so. As a result, their performance isn't exemplary – it's just good enough for them to keep their jobs.

(Of course, there are other contributing factors. People who suffer from depression, anxiety, arthritis, diabetes, high blood pressure and other ailments lose much of the productivity they once had.)

This epidemic of 'presenteeism' is spreading fast, and not just in the workforce. Technically, people might be present on the job – or with their families or when taking part in activities they once actively enjoyed – but they're not engaged, not thriving, not striving. They're bogged down with the demands of life, suffering from ailments, sleepwalking through their days with no light at the end of the tunnel. The thought of doing the same thing for the next 15 or 20 years, with no increase in quality of life, can be immobilizing: no wonder so many people suffer from depression. If you don't have a game plan to handle the demands of life, to create energy, you'll never lead the life you want to lead.

In the next chapter, we'll help you *rewire* your mindset so you can create *change* and develop *routines*, formulating great *habits* that will last a lifetime. Most diet and exercise programmes assume that if you eat right and get into better shape, everything else will take care of itself. Well, aside from a lucky (and dedicated) few, that only works for the short term, and most of us need a game plan to keep us going. After all, even the most physically gifted athletes cannot succeed unless they have mentally addressed everything they will face in competition. Developing the proper mindset will help prepare you for everything that comes your way.

MINDSET

NUTRITION

MOVEMENT

RECOVERY

NUTRITION

If you want to create that core Super Ball, you have to fuel your body properly. Even if you do nothing else (i.e., exercise), eating right will go a long way towards protecting your health.

I've never understood why diet books outsell fitness books by such a large margin. Apparently, more people would rather deprive themselves of food through dieting than take a proactive approach to their health through a combination of nutrition and exercise.

You won't find that here. What you *will* find is that together, we're going to change your approach to eating. Instead of living to eat, we're going to *eat to live*. It's that simple. Instead of using food to change your emotional state or deal with stress, you're going to use it to fuel your body for maximum performance. It's not just about losing weight or looking good in a bathing suit – both of which you'll accomplish, by the way.

Instead, you're going to use food to fuel your success and sustain your energy level. Not only that, but by planning to eat properly and putting a nutrition game plan in place, you'll also save yourself time and money.

MOVEMENT

I hesitate to use the term *exercise* because it's come to mean something with a definitive beginning and end: *I'm going to the gym now, so therefore it's time to exercise.*

I prefer the term *movement* since it's more indicative of an active lifestyle, even outside the gym. I'll show you ways to work your body in any situation, whether it's sitting at your desk or sitting in an aeroplane. It can be as simple as taking the stairs instead of the lift. Try to take every opportunity to move your body, not just during formal exercise. Think of your entire life as a potential workout.

Proper movement is what will give your 'Super Ball' its power; otherwise, you're more like a soft ball. There might be a solid core in there somewhere, but it's covered with so many layers of string that it has minimal impact. With this programme of proper exercise, you'll develop those 'super' powers.

RECOVERY

'I give 110 per cent every day.'

If I really meant that, I'd be lying. The reason I'd be lying is that nobody can give 110 per cent – or 100 per cent, for that matter – every day. The body, mind and soul won't allow it.

There are people who work 18-hour days, 6 days a week, and never take a holiday. What's the point? I know there are people who love their work – I'm fortunate to be one of them – but if I didn't have the time to enjoy the fruits of my labour then I'd be wasting my life.

Not just that, but it's impossible to maintain such a furious pace without your body breaking down. Throughout this programme, you'll learn the importance of recovery, or what I like to call *regeneration.*

A fast bowler in cricket, for instance, cannot bowl all day. He needs breaks. Yes, he can bowl for short stints during the day. But it's impossible for any bowler to go all-out all day without risking injury. Regeneration is necessary.

Regeneration applies to everything: exercise, nutrition and mindset. You can't work out hard 6 days a week; your body will break down. So, we've constructed this programme with hard days and easier 'regeneration days' that allow you time to recover.

The same is true with nutrition. If I instructed you to eat nothing but healthy foods, 7 days a week, you'd never be able to follow the programme. So I'm giving you one day a week to eat however you please. It allows you to take a mental break and reward yourself. (By the way, there's also a 3-week indoctrination period to help you to build up to eating healthy for most of the week.)

Regeneration also applies to your mindset. The primary purpose of a holiday is for your mind to recover from the grind of everyday life. We need to build these breaks into our lives in order to come back even stronger.

Think of how that Super Ball continues to bounce high six, seven or eight times. We want to bounce back from the demands and pitfalls of life, returning stronger each time. Recovery is the ability to come back up to that level as rapidly as possible. Recovery allows us to create constant momentum.

These four components – Mindset, Nutrition, Movement and Recovery – do not operate independently. This is an integrated programme that will permeate every aspect of your life. So let's begin with establishing that proper mindset.

Chapter 1 Summary: *Core Performance Essentials* is not just a diet and exercise programme but an integrated lifestyle system that incorporates the four elements of the Core Essentials sphere. Those components are Mindset, Nutrition, Movement and Recovery. By working on all four aspects of the system, you can produce the energy and structure to thrive in the Game of Life.

CHAPTER 2

THE CORE SELF

Most people end their work day with a false sense of accomplishment. They do a great job of playing goalie, handling tasks and juggling duties at a furious pace. At the end of the day, however, are they really better off? Have they invested in the long-term health of their bodies through physical activity and proper nutrition? Have they gone on the offensive, guided by core values, and worked towards personal goals that will bring about lasting change? Or have they merely endured another day of making a living?

Think of yourself for a moment as a powerful force for producing change in the lives of family and friends. What have you done each day to build your powers? Not just in your career, but in terms of making yourself into the person you want to be? What are the core values and goals that drive you?

Unlike in sport, the difference between winning and losing in this game is not always clear. How can it be if we haven't defined the rules we play by? Do we really know what will make us 'successful'? Do we let society dictate to us its view of success? Is it really about accumulating financial wealth, looking like a

THE MEANING OF SUCCESS

What is your definition of success?

What roles do you play at home, at work?

What drives you?

What would the other people you touch through your various roles say about you today, as opposed to what you'd like them to say about you in a eulogy?

What do you need to do in order to create the change so that they will say what you would like to hear in your eulogy?

magazine model or having the most friends on the block? Is it just about getting that next promotion, getting the children to their next appointment on time, losing those 5 kilograms (10 pounds) we swore we would? Or have we not truly examined what will mean everything to us when we look back on our lives?

We need to make a deeper examination. You have unique roles in life, and I'd venture to say that there is nobody out there who plays just one part. When an athlete comes to me, I need to know which sport and which position he plays before we even think about defining his goals and the success he hopes to attain. Without knowing what role he plays on his team, we can't accomplish anything together. Similarly, there are a lot of positions you could play. Through 'The Meaning of Success' and 'What Roles Do You Play in the Game of Life?' exercises described here, you are going to think about and define your positions and responsibilities in the game.

Once you've done this, we need to do the same thing that I do with superstar athletes: evaluate you, based on where you are and what you need to improve to perform your position well. And then, together, we'll create sustainable change that allows you to do a better job playing your various positions and supporting your team.

This process should change your mindset, giving you tangible goals based on who you are and whom you support, not on how much you make or how you look. Throughout this book, we'll give you the game plan that will help you live up to the high standards you should – and will – set for yourself. It will be the best investment of time you'll ever make. Take a moment now and create your own meaning of success through the exercise above. You can write in the book, but perhaps it would be more effective to use a separate sheet of paper that you can access more easily.

This is a deeply personal exercise, but my

advice for everyone is the same: dream big. For me, success is directly correlated with the depths of my relationships with the people I care about most. I will have been successful if I have helped to improve the quality of their lives. If I've done that, then my life will have stood for something special and will continue to live on in those people long after I'm gone.

My definition of success also would be to fully use what God and my parents gave me, to the best of my abilities, and to carry on those family values they taught me. Perhaps the biggest value I learnt growing up was the notion of service, to make sure that I lead by example in all areas of my life and to help others so that they can do the same. Through hard work, passion, honesty and the courage to lead the life that I've dreamed of, I can be-come successful. I will not accept anything less from myself.

Even if you've never defined success, I'm guessing deep down that you know what your vision of real accomplishment is and what you want to create. We all have core values that we do not want to compromise. Every day, we're faced with choices to make the right de-cisions, and it takes strength and courage to do that as you make your way towards your best self.

But you need to have that direction. For our purposes, it doesn't matter what your definition of success is – what's important is that it will point the way to fulfilment. This is your inspira-tion to get in the game.

Through the exercise below, ask yourself what you need to fulfil all of the roles you play.

WHAT ROLES DO YOU PLAY IN THE GAME OF LIFE?

What are your roles? What do you need to do for each of these roles? What will be the definition of success to improve quality in each one of these roles in life? Ask yourself:

What will make you feel successful in the areas of mental, physical and spiritual development?
What will make you feel successful in the important role you play for your spouse or partner?
What do you need to do to be successful in your role with your family?
What role do you fill with your friends? How can you fill this role more successfully?
What is your role with your colleagues at work, at college, in the organizations of which you're a part?

What role do you play for your spouse or partner? What roles do you play to make the relationship special? What does your position require? When discussing what they need to play their roles effectively on the field, athletes mention things like speed, strength and agility. When you're talking about making a relationship work, it's about listening and being understanding. It's about creating and spending meaningful time together.

Once you've defined the roles you play, ask yourself what other people would say about you in these roles. Would your spouse say that you don't make enough time, or that you are not intimate enough when you do? What would you want your spouse or partner to say?

What would your family say about you? Would parents or siblings say that you don't take the time to call? Would your children say that you don't have time to read a bedtime story? Perhaps they would say you're conscientious about making calls outside of birthdays and that you readily engage in random acts of kindness. You're the person they can turn to for advice, help or support.

What would your friends say about you? Would they say that you're there for them when they need you? Or would they say that they're tired of hearing about all your problems, about how life has been unfair? How about your colleagues? Would they say you're a nice person? Would they describe you as productive and

effective at work or as someone who drags down the office?

If you work in an office or go to college, would your colleagues say that you play around too much? Or have you found the happy medium, able to buckle down when you have to, but not taking yourself too seriously? Are you known for laughing and having fun or for being stressed out and holding on too tight?

In short, what do you want people to think or say about you? Go back to each of the roles listed above. Are you setting a good example? Are you comfortable with the way you're perceived by those around you?

So, what does any of this have to do with nutrition and exercise? In a word: everything. You need to identify these core values before you can embark on a physical transformation. It will give you added motivation to work towards your long-term success plan, but, more important, you'll come to recognize that this isn't just about you – you're undertaking this transformation to better serve and elevate the people you care about most.

The concept of being **guided by core values** in a programme of energy production, exercise and proper nutrition in the interest of achieving long-term success and elevating the lives of others is what I call the **centred self** or *core self*. Keep in mind that your core is the centre of your own world, but that doesn't mean that things revolve around you.

Instead, use that strong core to elevate others.

Sounds simple enough. Unfortunately, we've become such a self-centred culture that we fail to look inside ourselves, into our cores, for deeper meaning and guidance. Whatever happened to all that discussion after 9/11 about how we'd take a broader view of ourselves, strip away the superficial nonsense and focus on what's really important?

That didn't last long. Now we have the plague of reality television and extreme makeover shows promising immediate solutions for everything from our faces to our homes. We walk around with mobile phones glued to our ears, oblivious to everyone else. We're obsessed with six-pack abs, celebrity and overnight stardom. There are books and magazines devoted to 'trading up' in everything from clothes to cars to homes. We've created superstars out of people like Donald Trump and Paris Hilton, mostly for being rich and self-centred.

This might seem like a digression, but it speaks to the core (pun intended) of what we're trying to accomplish in this programme. If you look at your diet and exercise programme as just another quick-fix, must-have accessory or luxury item, this is not going to work in the long-term.

Among the many reasons why most nutrition and exercise programmes do not produce lasting change is that people view their health as something to be renovated, a remodelling project with a definitive beginning and end. They want the fastest, easiest possible solution, and, failing that, there's always plastic surgery and liposuction.

People tend to make changes from the outside in. But unless you make fundamental changes, overhauling your mindset, it's just short-term, until one day you wake up not quite sure who you are, where you've been or where you want to go.

Life isn't about finding yourself; it's about *creating* yourself. Who do you want to be? That's the great thing about sport. Children pretend they're someone else who plays a certain way. They grow up emulating the qualities and abilities that they like. That's how they shape their development – by mimicking the people who do it best.

We're all works in progress, and that process of *real* self-improvement should never stop. The biggest question any of us needs to answer is: *Who do you want to be, and why?* What's important to you? Is it family, friends and relationships? Is it exercise and staying active? If you had all the money in the world, what are the things you would do? What fulfils you?

Once we've defined success and considered the roles we play, it's easier to look at ourselves from the perspective of the **centred self as opposed to being self-centred**.

By embarking on this process, you're going to be better able to lift your friends and family, but it starts with you.

Understand that you're building from the inside out, mentally and physically. If you take care of that and work through this process to improve the quality of your life through both nutrition and exercise, then you'll be on your way towards real fulfilment – and that's what leads to lasting change.

It's the difference between being a show car and a racing car. You might see a racing car at a trade show or in a car showroom. It looks like a real racing car and has all the right fittings and decals, but actually there's nothing under the bonnet. The real racing car, with the high-performance engine and modern technology, is somewhere else.

Like that racing car, we want to build our core to perform for specific purposes, to sustain higher levels of energy and wellbeing. That's the type of person we're trying to build – not that empty shell of a show car.

The centred self is guided by deeper meaning, and it looks to elevate others. The self-centred person thinks, 'I just want to look better'. If that's the case, why not just get chest implants and liposuction? It's a lot less time-consuming than training.

As we've made clear, looking good isn't motivation enough to establish a long-term, life-changing game plan. You'll lose weight and look better, perhaps temporarily, but once that's accomplished, it will be tougher to motivate yourself to continue. But if you're working for a higher purpose, it's easier to focus on that as constant motivation.

You have to feel a deeper, emotional connection to your health; otherwise, it's just another project to complete and cross off the list. But if you can feel the changes that improved health produces, it will serve as constant motivation, whether it's the immediate endorphin rush after a workout, the sustained energy you feel all day long from eating correctly or the greater financial security you create for yourself and your loved ones.

But, of course, it's not enough to say, 'Okay, starting today, I'm going to be less self-centred and focus more on my core values and helping those who matter most to me.' That's not a bad mission statement, but you need to execute the strategy, driven by the exercises on pages 10 to 11. Otherwise, you'll just get caught up in the whirlwind of daily routines and end up playing goalie again. You either produce energy or you take it away, and if you take it away, you risk ending up as one of those 36 million people who die every year from illness related to obesity and inactivity.

Think of those examples from earlier in the book of the business executive on the corporate treadmill; the harried, stay-at-home parent; and the frazzled student. Or just look at yourself in the mirror. Take an inventory of how you're prematurely ageing. Besides the extra

'The Gift of Health'

NAME: MIKE DIXEY
AGE: 36
OCCUPATION: PHYSIOTHERAPIST

Mike Dixey's life was literally spiralling out of control. In 1999, he got out of bed after celebrating his birthday the night before, and he fell to the ground. The room was spinning. 'I wouldn't have been worried if I had been drinking,' Dixey says. 'But I don't drink.'

Over the next 5 months, Dixey underwent MRIs and CT scans and visited neurologists. He was diagnosed with vertigo, though doctors didn't know what was causing it.

'The only thing they knew was that my eyes were not seeing what my brain was registering,' Dixey says. 'Whenever I made a quick change of position, I'd have trouble. I'd wake up and the room would be spinning.'

And that was when he *could* sleep. Dixey spent nights tossing and turning, unable to fall into a restful sleep. Travelling on aeroplanes was difficult. He maintained a strict regime of medication. Doctors told him he would have to live with the condition for the rest of his life.

Because he was also dealing with the chaos of being a new father, getting up constantly at night to help with baby feedings and eating whenever and whatever he could, he put on 14 kilograms (about 30 pounds). Many nights, he ate pizza or Chinese takeaways at 10:30 p.m. or later.

Dixey knew that he was a heart attack waiting to happen, what with a long history of heart disease in his family. His father has survived a heart attack and his mother, triple-bypass surgery. Three aunts underwent quadruple bypasses. Dixey's paternal grandfather died young from a heart attack.

Throughout his twenties, he had worked out using bodybuilding-style routines. That did little to change his overall fitness, and he underwent knee surgery and suffered from back and shoulder pain. 'I never realized that I had reached a plateau long ago,' he says. 'I wasn't seeing any benefit.'

It's not that Dixey didn't understand the challenge; he works as a physiotherapist and has a vast library of fitness literature. In 2004, he began the Core programme, eating properly and performing movement-based exercises.

'It's the first programme I had found that combined flexibility, strength and rotator cuff movements. Everything about it made so much more sense.'

Dixey lost 9.5 kilograms (21 pounds) in the first 12 weeks of the programme and dropped 14.5 kilograms (32 pounds) overall. Soon his back, shoulders and knees were pain-free. He was able to touch his toes for the first time since childhood, and he made plans to play in the local cricket team.

Most importantly, the vertigo all but disappeared. He still feels a mild form occasionally if he is stuck in traffic with cars whizzing by from the other side. But he's off medication and sleeping peacefully – or at least as well as any parent with two children under the age of 6 can expect.

'I look great, and more important, I feel great,' Dixey says. 'I'm looking forward to playing cricket and being back in control of my life. That's the greatest gift this programme has given me – the gift of great health.'

kilos, you're dehydrated, which ages the skin more. You have poor posture from sitting so much and not exercising, so you look slouched over, older and less confident. Since you don't get enough sleep, you have bags under your eyes, get sick more often, have less energy and look perpetually run-down. You find it increasingly difficult to concentrate and be productive at work. Perhaps you're on medication, or you self-medicate with alcohol or drugs, which only exacerbates your problems. No doubt your sex drive isn't what it once was.

I know you mean well. Against all of these odds, you've been successful at work and at home, to one degree or another. In a sense, you've sacrificed your body for the good of the team, your loved ones. You're doing everything possible to be that centred self. But if

you don't make immediate changes to reverse this downward spiral, your team is going to suffer some big-time losses.

Think of someone you know who has died young from a heart attack or an illness brought about by an unhealthy lifestyle. Maybe this person had it all – wealth, family, an enviable career. But none of it means anything because they couldn't stay around to affect the lives of others.

You can't buy health, which is vital to becoming a centred self. By placing a premium on relationships, core values and long-term goals that elevate others, you come to the conclusion that health is the vehicle that drives the system.

It's impossible to accomplish anything without health. If you're constantly tired, run-down and playing goalie, unable to take care of

DETERMINATION

CONSISTENCY

TEAMWORK

yourself, how can you ever think about others? It even breeds resentment to the point that you might think, 'I'm killing myself here and nobody appreciates it!'

We need to learn to be better teammates. Here's where we can learn from professional athletes: they can inspire us with their dedication to the team and, every so often, to a much higher cause.

Let's consider three concepts from sport that apply:

Sport, at its essence, is people overcoming obstacles. Athletes have the **determination** to stare down adversity with unwavering confidence in themselves, whether it's a tennis player who is two sets down and comes back to win the match, or a football team that wins the game having been 2–0 at half time.

Athletes reap the rewards in the form of great fame and fortune. You toil more anonymously, trying each day to reach your goals and realize your aspirations. Regardless, like a world-class athlete, you have to stay steadfastly focused on your goals, and you have to remain confident that you can attain them. At the end of the day, you have to ask yourself if you've moved closer – even by just a few centimetres – to achieving a specific goal.

The key is to be consistent. **Consistency** can be a misleading term since it's often associated with repetition, complacency and mediocrity. But for our purposes, look at it as the consistent pursuit of greatness. After all, there are plenty of recreational golfers who can play one round on a PGA course and shoot a 68. But can they do it consistently? That's the difference between world-class performance and having a good day. Great golfers have become so consistent that even on their worst days, they're still pretty damned good. When you can sustain that high level of performance and build upon it over the course of a career, that's when you achieve true greatness.

We want to take that same approach to our health, especially in the workouts we'll discuss later in the book. We don't aspire to consistent mediocrity, so that we end up complacent and doing the same routines over and over, never getting better, just getting bored. We want to seek consistent greatness.

Teamwork is perhaps the greatest motivating factor in establishing that consistency. Even in individual sports such as tennis and golf, athletes have a small army of supporters. There are coaches and trainers, family and friends, and all manner of support staff.

Being part of a team carries an enormous responsibility. You never want to be viewed as the weakest link or as letting your teammates down. Instead, you want to raise the level of play and achievement of the entire team, regardless of your position.

Even if you don't play any sport, you're a

member of at least one team: your immediate family. Perhaps you've reached the point where you've spun off and formed an expansion team, a family of your own.

Those are important teams, and you must play your position extremely well in order to support those around you and get the most out of the game of life. That means you have to be a little selfish in finding time to take care of your body. This is where a lot of people go wrong: they rationalize eating poorly, working longer hours and failing to exercise by thinking they are doing it for their loved ones. 'I don't have time to exercise or eat right. I must forge ahead and work harder. My family is counting on me!'

It sounds almost heroic. But though your intentions are good, you're actually letting down the team. It's like the guy who tries to continue playing his sport on a dodgy ankle or knee, getting by at 50 per cent. It's impressive, and sometimes adequate, but sooner or later he's going to break down, and he'll bring the team down with him.

The same holds true in life. If you have struggled in the past with nutrition and exercise, it's time to start thinking of the impact on your most important team. Professional athletes get replaced all the time. There's always another player out there who's younger, faster, cheaper, and so players get released, they get traded, and eventually hang up their boots. But you're an irreplaceable part of your team.

So, in order to make sure you can be there for your team, let's start by properly fuelling your body, the vehicle for your success. We'll start in the next section with the Core Nutrition programme – everything you need to know to maintain a high-performance, healthy diet. Though the nutrition section comes before the workout, I don't mean to imply that one is more important than the other, though I understand why some people place more importance on eating right than working out. After all, everyone has to eat to survive, so why not just diet, rather than spending time and effort working out? People figure they don't *have* to exercise to lose weight, though it's pretty tough to live a healthy lifestyle on just diet alone. You get so much more benefit out of a nutritional programme if you exercise as well – and vice versa. Remember that what and how you eat is only *part of* building your centred self.

In fact, you'll find that when you combine a proper nutritional programme with a core-based workout that emphasizes functional movement, you'll be in a position to accomplish almost anything. You'll be fitter, healthier and ready to face any challenge

I've made the workout programme in this book as easy and time-sensitive as possible, but if you find that there are times when you can't follow it, whether that's because you are too busy, or you are unwell, then just stick to the nutrition portion. That alone will improve your health significantly. But let's make this a perfect progression: you established your core values and centred self in this section. Now, let's change our eating habits and create a workout programme that will maximize our future success.

Throughout this book, you'll hear from people who managed to do just that by following the Core Performance programme.

Chapter 2 Summary: Successful people are driven by core values that permeate every fibre of their being. By defining success through these values and applying it to each of the roles you play in life, it's possible to accomplish just about anything. Unlike many people in our self-centred society, we each want to be a centred self, or core-centred, using these values as fuel for our daily lives and our long-term goals.

MINDSET

NUTRITION

MOVEMENT

RECOVERY

CORE
NUTRITION

CHAPTER 3

TWO-MINUTE WARNING

You might think nutrition doesn't matter. Maybe you've got along just fine with a little extra weight. Unfortunately, the older you get, the more those surplus kilos take their toll. You're more vulnerable to heart disease and diabetes, you have less energy and you don't accomplish as much as you otherwise could. No matter how successful you are, I'm sure you'll agree that you could do even more if you were in better shape.

The bottom line is that, left unchecked, your body is a crisis waiting to happen. Consider this your two-minute warning. Fortunately, there's still time. In the same way as some professional athletes have managed to fashion a record-breaking career from a last-minute comeback, we're going to show you how to turn your nutrition plan around quickly.

Maybe you already have a good plan in place. At this point, you have a game plan to build your centred self. You've installed an athlete's mentality and know to build everything from the core. But think of yourself as the general manager of a new franchise with far greater resources.

Now we're going to literally transform our

bodies through nutrition. You will learn how to eat and drink to fuel your body for optimal energy and production. In short, the Core Nutrition game plan is a great way to maximize energy, lose fat, gain lean mass and save money and time.

But before you get started with the programme, please complete the Core Nutrition Assessment above.

The purpose behind these questions is to illustrate that at the core of great nutrition are *environment* and *planning,* things as simple as the power of your cupboards, fridge, freezer and a well-stocked desk at work. So, if you answered no to either of the first two questions and yes to either of the last two questions in the Core Nutrition Assessment, you're setting yourself up for long-term health problems.

As with the rest of this programme, I want you to think like an athlete about nutrition. After all, you're certainly competing in a high-stakes game, and you need a powerful, turbocharged body that burns fuel efficiently and produces the consistent energy you'll need to reach your full potential.

If you consume fizzy drinks, burgers and fast food regularly, you'll end up among the ranks of the obese, putting yourself at an extreme disadvantage in everything you do. Oh, you don't agree? Well, in 2003, filmmaker Morgan Spurlock tried to eat nothing but McDonald's for an entire month. A healthy, fit young man when he started, he put on more than 9 kilograms (20 pounds) in a couple of weeks. Soon he was walking around in a daze, with little energy and an addiction to the food. His doctors and nutritionists told him that if he did not stop the McDonald's diet, his vital organs might shut down and his health could be permanently damaged.

Spurlock's movie, *Super Size Me,* inspired McDonald's to eliminate its largest portions from its menu. He deserves praise for educating the public on the dangers of fast food and how it's so shamelessly marketed.

We're up against the wall when it comes to eating properly. Everywhere we turn, someone's trying to sell us quick, convenient, cheap junk food. They will stop at nothing, labelling food 'low fat' or 'low carb', even as they load it up with high-fructose corn syrup and trans fats, two fat-producing substances we'll discuss in-depth later.

From now on, be an educated consumer when it comes to playing the food game. Be a smart player. Whether it's taking time to consider the healthy options when ordering a restaurant meal or reading a label for contents, you need to make the best decision for your healthy lifestyle, which you'll learn how to do in the next chapters.

Most importantly, you have to plan and prepare. Otherwise, you're at the mercy of what's out there, most of which is not good. The number one reason people don't eat properly and sabotage their fitness programmes is because of sloppy planning.

When it comes to nutrition, like everything else in this programme, you have to think for the long term. It's easy to rationalize eating unhealthy food – after all, you're hungry and you need to eat something. You're not *that* overweight. Perhaps you didn't want to be rude to your hosts, refusing that high-fat dish they served. Besides, it really tastes good!

Each time you face such a dilemma, stop and ask why you're on the brink of eating whatever junk food is at hand. Are you letting emotions drive your decisions? What could you do to make a better decision? Even if you are stuck in a fast-food restaurant, what's the best choice available?

After all, those few moments of junk-food-induced pleasure end quickly. So, too, does the value of the food in terms of producing energy. Soon you'll be hungry again. There's also the negative long-term impact that the unhealthy food will have on your body.

Make a positive investment instead. Each time you eat properly, remind yourself that you're not only giving yourself the energy needed for optimal performance, but you're also investing in your long-term health – to say nothing of helping yourself feel and look better than you ever have before.

I know the prospect of embarking on a new nutrition plan is scary. Maybe you've tried other diets. You've counted calories or carbs, followed the Atkins or Zone diets – whichever one happens to be trendy this week. Perhaps you've experimented with miracle supplements that supposedly help you to lose weight or gain energy. None of them have proved to be a complete, long-term solution. Instead, they set you up for failure.

The challenge with most programmes is that they tend to address the symptoms – too much weight and a lack of energy – rather than the problem, which is poor nutrition in general.

Under this plan, you're going to have five or six small meals or snacks a day, which means you get to eat something every 2½ to 3 hours. If you eat often, your body becomes a more efficient energy-producing machine. (Ask yourself what burns more wood, a hot fire or smouldering coals?) Not only that, frequent eating keeps you from overeating. If you know you're going to have something more to eat in a few hours, you'll be less likely to overeat now – and less likely to be extremely hungry.

The reason most people don't eat properly is because they don't plan ahead. Remember the athletic mentality? If an athlete does not prepare, looking ahead to what he will face in the game, he's doomed to fail. The same is true with eating. If you don't plan ahead and stock up on nutritious foods, you end up devouring whatever you can grab.

The process of stressing out over where and when to eat is unhealthy, a problem made worse by the junk you inevitably consume in such a state. As a result, you end up increasing body fat and decreasing lean mass, which defeats the purpose of following the Core Movement programme in the next section. Not only that, but eating on the run is more expensive than eating to the Core Nutrition plan. It costs more, not just in terms of the money

you lay out at the restaurant, but in terms of the damage it does to your health.

As we formulate our game plan, let's take a look at the strengths of our opponent, which really aren't strengths at all but widely held misconceptions about nutrition.

Eating right is time-consuming: On the contrary, eating right saves time. If you have your meals plotted out for the entire day – or the entire week – you'll save hours of shopping and preparation time each week.

Compare the person in your office who brings lunch from home with the person who has to go out to a sit-down restaurant, an unhealthy fast-food franchise or a sandwich shop. The one who brought lunch from home already has saved a minimum of 15 to 30 minutes of their lunch hour, and most probaby he'll eat a healthier lunch as well.

I'm not advocating eating at your desk, though in many hectic offices this is reality. If that's the case, and your don't bring your lunch from home, you'll fall behind by popping out to buy lunch. Not only that, but if you have lunch handy, you're less likely to go hungry and rush out to find the first option available. One easy way to get a jump start on the week's food preparation is to do all your shopping on Saturdays or Sundays, which will help you to plan out your meals for the week. This is a great way to be really proactive about making healthy choices.

'I proved the drug company rep wrong.'

NAME: PAT BINKLEY

AGE: 36

OCCUPATION: SOFTWARE EXECUTIVE

Like a lot of new parents, Pat Binkley struggled to find the time to exercise. With a hectic schedule as an executive for a software company and three children under the age of 6, he saw no openings in his schedule.

Still, he knew he had to find a way. His cholesterol was 7. He carried 77 kilograms (170 pounds) on his 1.75-metre (5-foot-9 frame), which, although hardly obese, 'was bad weight', according to Binkley. 'I had a double chin and a pretty good spare tyre going. I even had man boobs.'

Binkley joined a gym, began leaving home at 5:30 for morning workouts, and followed the Core programme religiously. He made it home to shower and have breakfast before the children got out of bed.

'There was no way I was going to find an hour in the day anywhere else,' Binkley says of his early mornings. 'I'm sort of a morning person anyway. I had to do it. Now it's become my sacred time.'

Binkley overhauled his diet. He began looking at the supermarket in terms of zones, focusing on the outer aisles, where produce, meats and healthier foods are kept. He learnt how to study labels for nutrition content. Most important, he made sure he snacked on the right kinds of food throughout the day.

'I'm more aware now that I can't let my body go into starvation mode,' he says. 'I try to eat something during those long in-between periods. That gives me more consistent energy all day long and allows me to eat less during what used to be three larger meals. If you don't have those in-between-meal snacks, you're going to make poor decisions and overeat later.'

Since starting the programme in March 2004, Binkley has felt stronger. The spare tyre has begun to disappear. His wife has noticed the difference. Then there are the intangible rewards: 'The thing that surprised me the most is how much more energy I have for the children,' he says. 'I can pick them up and even hold two or three of them at a time. Before, my back would be hurting. Now I can put the heaviest child up on my shoulders. I can wrestle with them, ride bikes, play catch – be there for all of those quality-time things that I couldn't really enjoy before.'

These days, Binkley's weight is down to a lean 71 kilograms (157 pounds). His cholesterol is staying down below 5. He recently ran into a drug company rep who once told him that it was impossible to reduce cholesterol by more than 10 per cent – let alone 35 – by diet and exercise alone.

'I thought I'd need [to take] drugs,' Binkley says. 'I still wonder if I'm going to be able to make this a lifelong routine as opposed to something I did for a couple of years in my mid-thirties. But when you feel good and can be there for your children, that's all the motivation you need.'

Eating right is expensive: Actually, eating right *saves* money. If you've planned your day and week, chances are you'll eat out infrequently, which saves a lot of cash. When you have not prepared ahead of time – like the re-active office worker above – you're more likely to grab the first option available when you're hungry, regardless of cost.

Let's not forget the greater cost of eating out: the cost to your health. Researchers at the University of Massachusetts in the United States found that eating more than one-third of your meals in restaurants increases your risk of obesity by 69 per cent.

Eating right means I'll only be consuming bland, tasteless food: This is a big misconception. It's easy to prepare meals that not only are good for you but that also taste good. There are dozens of delicious foods, condiments and spices that we'll discuss in the coming pages that will help you to prepare and eat meals that are both healthy and delicious.

Fast-food restaurants thrive because they perpetuate all these myths. After all, they provide tasty, inexpensive food, quickly. That food might be cheap, though it's still not as inexpensive as planning and preparing your own meals at home. Moreover, low-nutrient, high-sugar, high-fat foods rob us of energy, produce nasty mood swings that affect our relationships and our decision-making abilities, and increase body fat. In the long term, this may decrease your qual-ity of life and overall well-being, as well as your life expectancy.

We have come to believe that, even though we work hard, we have no control over our lives and are not able to make the most of our potential. It's a brutal downward spiral. We end up making the excuses that there's not enough time to exercise and prepare healthy meals, that we're in too much pain, that we don't have enough energy or that spending time with family is more important than taking time to plan and stick to a healthy game plan.

It all starts with the food we eat. No matter how diligently we follow the Core Workout – or any exercise programme – it won't matter unless we properly fuel our bodies with the right kinds of foods and nutrients.

Did you know that most people eat poorly 80 per cent of the time and healthily the remaining 20 per cent? Most of the time, they consume high-calorie foods that are low in nutrients and fibre.

We want to flip that equation, striving to eat healthily at least 80 per cent of the time. It's unrealistic to think that we'll be perfect, no matter how hard we plan. Plus, we're building in a 'free' day to eat whatever you want each week, within reason. That's one-seventh of a week right there.

So, let's sound the two-minute warning. No longer will we be nutritional goalies, scooping up everything that comes our way with little thought for how it affects our health and wellbeing. Instead, we're going to deflect these shots, letting in only those foods that will fuel us well, provide energy and contribute to long-term health.

Chapter 3 Summary: The key to eating properly is planning. By stocking the cupboards, fridge and freezer with healthy options at home, you avoid eating poorly at home. By keeping an office cabinet supplied with similar foods, you avoid having to grab caffeinated drinks or snacks at the vending machine to keep you going. Eating healthy meals and snacks saves money and time, and can also save your health in the long term.

CHAPTER 4

REVIEWING THE RULE BOOK

W e've become accustomed to eating a certain way because, well, that's the way it's always been. We accept certain nutrition rules as inalienable truths when many of them are misconceptions. In this chapter, we're going to review and rewrite the rule book, inserting new strategies that will properly fuel our bodies and give us energy to really live.

CORE NUTRITION STRATEGY 1: EAT OFTEN

We've been taught to eat three square meals a day, avoid between-meal snacks and not eat after dinner. No wonder we tend to feel bloated from overeating, hungry and lethargic between meals, and starved before bedtime.

To control appetite, regulate your blood sugar level (which improves concentration and helps to regulate appetite) and build lean body mass, you must eat five or six small- to medium-size meals or snacks each day. That means you need to eat, on average, every 3 hours. Think of yourself as 'grazing' throughout the day, instead of sitting down for three massive meals as in the past.

Frequent eating is like constantly throwing wood on the fire. Digesting food cranks up your metabolism and burns more calories every time you eat. When you eat only occasionally, the fire smoulders and dies. A hot fire, on the other hand, burns wood continuously.

You can eat six times a day regardless of your job or lifestyle. The six 'meals' are not going to be long, sit-down affairs. Three of your meals could be a piece of fruit and a handful of nuts. Take what you might have previously considered a large lunch and save part of it for mid-afternoon.

On the days you work out, which might be every weekday, you'll consume pre- and/or post-workout recovery shakes. And since you're eating more often, your traditional breakfasts, lunches and dinners should be lighter.

If we don't eat often, the most readily available substance for the body to consume is muscle. Many people believe that the first thing the body eats away is fat. But that's a misconception – in point of fact, the body is remarkably resistant to fat loss and will turn to its lean muscle mass first, keeping that stored fat in reserve as long as necessary.

Many people try to get thin by not eating. They deprive their bodies of nutrients and, while they might look healthy, they may have dangerous blood profiles and a high ratio of fat to lean muscle. Their bodies are what I call 'skinny fat' (others call them 'skinny soft'). They look skinny, but they actually have a high percentage of body fat.

The last thing we want to do is lose lean mass. After all, we're going to be working hard to build this lean mass, which produces power, stabilizes joints, promotes movement and is critical for optimal performance. We lose half a kilogram of lean mass per year after our mid-twenties, so it's imperative to take action to maintain this lean mass and function.

To that end, we must eat often, which brings us to our next strategy . . .

CORE NUTRITION STRATEGY 2: CONTROL THE GAME CLOCK

Everyone has a different schedule. But like a good football, rugby or hockey team, we're going to use the clock to our advantage.

Here are three ways to schedule your six meals, depending on whether you work out in the morning, during lunch or after work. I've also included some menu suggestions and a schedule for those who compete in early evening sport.

Option A: For Those Who Work Out Before Work/College

6.15 a.m.

Pre-workout shooter (See '"Shot Clock" Pre- and Post-Exercise Nutrition' on pages 36 to 37.)

6.30 a.m.–7.30 a.m.

Workout

7.30 a.m.

Meal 1 (**Breakfast:** Egg-white omelette with vegetables)

10.30 a.m.

Meal 2 (Shake or snack)

1.30 p.m.

Meal 3 (**Lunch:** Tuna with low-fat mayonnaise

and/or celery, lettuce and tomato on whole-meal bread, or as a salad)

4.00 p.m.–4.30 p.m.

Meal 4 (Shake or snack)

7.00 p.m.–7.30 p.m.

Meal 5 (**Dinner:** Grilled salmon with vegetables and couscous)

10.00 p.m.–10.30 p.m.

Meal 6 (Shake or snack)

Option B: For Those Who Work Out during Lunch Hour

7.00 a.m.

Meal 1 (**Breakfast:** Porridge and a *small* piece of cold meat)

10.00 a.m.

Meal 2 (Shake or snack)

11.45 a.m.

Pre-workout shooter

Noon–1.00 p.m.

Workout

1.00 p.m.

Meal 3 (**Lunch:** Chicken breast on wholemeal bread with vegetables)

4.00 p.m.

Meal 4 (Shake or snack)

7.00 p.m.

Meal 5 (**Dinner:** A grilled cut of lean red meat with brown or wild rice and vegetables)

10.00 p.m.

Meal 6 (Shake or snack)

Option C: For Those Who Work Out after Work

7.00 a.m.

Meal 1 (**Breakfast:** A bowl of wholegrain cereal such as Kashi or shredded wheat with blueberries)

10.00 a.m.

Meal 2 (Shake or snack)

1.00 p.m.

Meal 3 (**Lunch:** Chicken breast on a bed of spinach or lettuce with sliced tomatoes, a small sprinkling of nuts and olive oil for dressing)

4.00 p.m.

Meal 4 (Shake or snack)

5.30 p.m.–6.30 p.m.

Workout

6.30 p.m.

Meal 5 (**Dinner:** Lean pork coated in wholemeal breadcrumbs seasoned with garlic, salt, pepper and mustard powder and a little oil with vegetables)

9.30 p.m.

Meal 6 (Shake or snack)

Option D: For Those Who Work Out or Compete in the Early Evening

7.00 a.m.

Meal 1 (**Breakfast:** Low-fat, low-sugar yogurt with flaxseed (linseed) oil and/or porridge)

10.00 a.m.

Meal 2 (Shake or snack)

1.00 p.m.

Meal 3 (**Lunch:** Lean turkey on rye, pumpernickel or sourdough bread with vegetables or a salad)

4.00 p.m.

Meal 4 (Shake or snack)

6.00 p.m.

Meal 5 (**Light dinner:** Seasoned grilled swordfish fillet with vegetables)

7.00 p.m.

Workout/Game/Competition

9.00 p.m.–9.30 p.m.

Meal 6 (Post-workout shake or snack)

This might seem as if you're eating a lot, but you're not, if you consume smaller portions. We've become accustomed to eating large servings. Fast-food restaurants now refer to them as 'value' sizes, to make you feel good about getting more for your money, even though you're still pigging out on junk.

One of the best ways to avoid overeating and maintain a healthy metabolism is to pay attention to portion sizes. By eating smaller portions more often, you give your body a better chance to digest and get all of the nutrients from the food. A piece of fish or meat should be about the size of a pack of cards, and a serving of starches (rice or pasta, for example) should be the size of a cricket ball. On the other hand, it's hard to eat too many vegetables.

Here's one simple way to eat the proper portions: use a smaller plate. Who says you have to use a huge plate as if you're loading up at an all-you-can-eat buffet? We've grown accustomed to thinking that we're not eating a full meal unless we fill up a big plate. By using a smaller one, it's easier to eat the proper portion.

Most people eat dinner around 7.00 p.m. and don't eat again until breakfast. That's as much as 12 hours without food, so your body gets through this extended fast by tapping into your lean muscle for nourishment. But, if you have that last snack at 10.00 p.m. and breakfast at 6.00 a.m., you can minimize the effects of the fast while getting a full night's sleep.

That final snack or shake at 10.00 p.m. should include something high in protein, since that helps to build lean muscle. You also want fibre and essential fats (such as those found in fish or flaxseed/linseed oil). For many people, a shop-bought protein shake or high-protein meal-replacement bar might be an easy option. Fruit with lean protein and healthy fat is another good choice that's easy to prepare, since fruit is full of antioxidants and can help to jump-start the body's regenerative process. So an ideal bedtime snack could be a protein shake with a teaspoon of flaxseed (linseed) oil and a handful of blueberries. Or perhaps try a glass of skimmed milk and a handful of almonds.

The bottom line is that by eating every 2½

to 3 hours, you'll maintain consistent energy levels and turn your body into an efficient, fat-burning machine.

CORE NUTRITION STRATEGY 3: BUILDING 'REAL DEAL' MEALS

When planning meals, it's vital to consider the role of carbohydrates, proteins, fats and fibre. Contrary to popular belief, they all must be included in an effective nutrition plan.

Carbs are our fuel, though the amount consumed must be proportional to your level of activity. If I fill up my car's petrol tank, drive 8 kilometres (5 miles) and then fill it up again, it's going to overflow. But, unlike with a car, you might not realize you're overfilling your tank and contributing to a higher level of body fat.

Generally speaking, the more active you are, the more carbs you want to consume. Since most people tend to be more active in the morning and afternoon, it makes sense to eat the majority of your carbs earlier in the day.

Every meal should include fruits and vegetables because of their fibre and nutrient densities. I recommend that you 'eat a rainbow often', which refers not only to the bright colours of fruits and vegetables but also to the fact that you should eat six small meals and snacks a day. Typically, your plate should consist mostly of colourful, high-fibre vegetables. There should be a piece of meat or fish (or a soya dish, if you are a vegetarian) the size of a pack of cards, and, if you like, a fist-size portion of

brown rice or wholewheat pasta. There also should be some 'good' fats in the form of, say, salmon or olive oil. (We'll discuss fats in more detail later in this chapter.)

When in doubt, remember to 'come back to Earth' – given a choice between something processed and something organic, go with the non-processed option.

Scouting Report: Carbs

Strengths: Provide energy for muscle function and act as the primary fuel for the brain. Some carbs, such as whole grains, fruits and vegetables, are rich in fibre, helping to control appetite, slow digestion and improve the health of your heart. Fruits and vegetables contain powerful antioxidants, helping to protect the body from the cell-damaging effects of free radicals.

Weaknesses: Processed carbs, such as white breads, pastas and baked goods, provide little nutritional value and are converted quickly to sugar and easily stored as fat.

Ideal Players:

● Fruits and Vegetables: apples, asparagus, aubergines (eggplants), avocados, beetroot, black beans, blackberries, blueberries, broccoli, brussels sprouts, cantaloupe, carrots, celery, cherries, cucumber, field greens, grapefruit, green apples, green beans, green peas, honeydew, kiwi fruit, mangoes, mushrooms, oranges, papaya, peaches, peppers (capsicums), pineapple, plums, pomegranates, raspberries, red

'SHOT CLOCK' PRE- AND POST-EXERCISE NUTRITION

You never want your body to be deprived of key nutrients, especially when you work out. Yet many people exercise first thing in the morning on an empty stomach. Don't get me wrong; exercising is a great way to start the day. But eat something before your workout, even if it's just half an apple or a pre-workout 'shooter', which is something like a watered-down glass of orange juice with a scoop of whey protein or simply a glass of water with the scoop of whey.

Whey gets into your system quickly, which is especially important for eating prior to or immediately following a workout. I also recommend a post-workout recovery shake. Most prepackaged shakes contain an effective ratio of proteins, carbohydrates and fat, and are loaded with fibre, vitamins and minerals. Since the shakes can be made by mixing water with a scoop or packet of powder in a covered plastic container or blender, they make a quick, easy and portable snack that won't spoil.

Ideally, you should have a shake right after the workout. At that point, your cells are wide open and screaming for nutrients, and by drinking one of these shakes, you expedite the recovery process and maximize the lean-muscle growth.

Recent research has also shown that the pre-workout shooter may produce an effect equal to a traditional post-workout recovery shake. The pre-workout shooter works its way into the bloodstream to give the muscle exactly what it needs at the earliest possible moment.

Everyone is different, so there's no one-size-fits-all routine I can offer. But if you remember the priorities – eating often and incorporating a pre-workout shooter and/or a post-workout recovery shake or meal – you can plan your day accordingly. (I'll even customize this to your exact schedule at our Web site, *www.coreperformance.com*)

SCOUTING REPORT: (WHEY) PROTEIN SHAKES

Strengths: A by-product of cheese manufacturing, whey includes many essential amino acids that boost the immune system and promote overall good health.

Weaknesses: None.

Ideal Players: Whey protein is found in post-workout recovery mixes, so you will be getting them in your shooters, but you also might

---

grapes, romaine lettuce, soyabeans, spinach, strawberries, sweet potatoes, tomatoes, watermelon, yams

● Breads, Cereals and Grains: Brown rice, couscous, oats, quinoa, rye bread, sourdough bread, wholemeal bread

Bottom Line: Non-processed, fibre–rich, colourful carbs are essential to a healthy lifestyle. Eliminating carbs produces sluggishness, along with long-term negative health effects. Carbohydrates are your fuel and should be consumed in proportion to your level of activity. Remember: a portion of carbs should be about the size of a baseball.

want to try adding an extra serving to your diet. The flavoured powder tastes great sprinkled on porridge or mixed with milk, water or juice.

Bottom Line: Whey provides numerous health benefits for a small investment of time and money.

Whey is quickly digested, which makes it great for eating around workouts. Many protein shakes combine whey protein with another type of slower-releasing protein, casein. This mixture provides a combination of fast- and slow-releasing proteins, which allows for complete coverage over the 2½- to 3-hour window between meals.

Protein shakes accelerate workout recovery. You can buy pre-made shakes, or you can make them yourself by mixing water with a scoop of powder. They're a quick and easy snack that's rich in lean protein but devoid of bad fats.

I recommend Myoplex, which is available online and from health food shops, a whey shake made by EAS. In the interest of full disclosure, let me say that EAS is one of my company's strategic partners. Could you get the same value in similar products from other manufacturers? Perhaps, though I've been in this business for more than 15 years and I've yet to find more effective products. Not only that, but EAS was also the first company to meet the stringent 'accuracy in labelling' standards of the NSF (National Sanitation Foundation, a US organization) and the 'banned-substance free' certification standards of the National Football League (NFL) and the NFL Players Association in the United States. I'm also a big fan of Amino Vital products. Yes, they're another one of my company's strategic partners, but I daresay that no other sports drink products on the market so effectively deliver the amino acids your body needs for higher performance. Amino Vital products are available online.

PRE-WORKOUT SHOOTER IDEAS
Either of these 'recipes' will provide a great pre-workout boost.

- 120 ml (4 fl oz) orange juice + 240 ml (8 fl oz) water + 1 scoop whey protein
- 1 scoop EAS Endurathon + 180–350 ml (6–12 fl oz) water

Bottom Line: Always have a post-workout shake or meal with carbohydrates and protein to aid recovery. Add a pre-workout shooter to speed up your recovery even more.

Low-Carb Diets

If you go on one of those diets without carbs, it's like taking a sponge and wringing the water out. You'll lose the water weight, but as soon as you eat carbs again – and you will at some point, because you need energy to function, and you can only go so long without carbs – then that sponge is going to fill up with water. Research shows that the weight will come right back, and with a vengeance; people often gain back all the weight they lost while following a diet that severely reduces carb intake – and more. As with all dieting, you'll probably lose some of your lean mass in the process.

Overall, carbs are an important part of your diet when you consume them relative to your activity level and within the context of the glycaemic index and glycaemic load, which we'll address below.

EVALUATING CARBOHYDRATE 'SPEED' WITH THE GLYCAEMIC INDEX STOPWATCH

Popular diets have brainwashed millions into believing that carbs are bad, full stop. If something is high in carbs, don't eat it.

Actually, carbs are essential for healthy living. Good carbs provide energy and are rich in fibre, and many are packed with powerful protective antioxidants.

So how can we tell the good carbs from the bad? Let's start with the *glycaemic index,* which is a measure of how a single food will raise your blood glucose level. For instance, let's compare broccoli with candy floss. If you eat 100 empty calories of candy floss, it dissolves quickly in your mouth and is absorbed immediately, sending your blood sugar level sky-high. Give children a high-glycaemic food such as candy floss, and they'll bounce off the walls. Even adults feel a sugar rush.

The problem is that you crash quickly and end up feeling sluggish. Your body then craves more sugar. Candy floss, not surprisingly, has a very high glycaemic index number.

If you eat 100 calories of nutrient-dense broccoli, however, your body will have to work much harder to break it down. Eating raw or slightly cooked broccoli (which retains its crunch) causes you to really *chew* it, while your mouth releases powerful digestive enzymes to help initiate the breakdown before the broccoli hits your stomach. It's going to take your body more time to digest. The benefit is that the sugar from the food will be released into your bloodstream more slowly, giving you steady energy over a longer period. In addition, fibre-rich broccoli sates your hunger and will, ahem,

keep things moving through your system. Broccoli, therefore, has a low glycaemic index number.

As a result, you should eat foods with low or moderate ratings on the glycaemic index. But since we rarely eat just one food at a time, we need to think about the body's overall glycaemic response to everything on our plates. If you eat a high-glycaemic food at the same time as some low-glycaemic foods, the overall *glycaemic response* is moderate, which is fine.

Another way to think of this is in terms of the glycaemic load (GL) of foods. GL takes into account both the quantity of the food to be consumed and how quickly the food raises blood sugar levels. GL looks at the amount of carbohydrate contained in an average serving of a food and uses this to calculate the overall affect that eating that food manufacturers removed fat from their products. Instead, some added additional high-fructose corn syrup into it to make up for the appealing taste that the fat had provided. This was a particularly common practice in the US.

Weaknesses: The reduced fat and added sugar in foods high in HFCS send blood sugar sky-high before crashing quickly. This process makes us hungry for more food, and so we will probably exceed our total caloric needs.

has on the body's blood sugar levels. This can give a fairly accurate indication of how the food will affect blood sugar levels.

Generally speaking, the lower the number on the glycaemic index, the more natural the food will be. Your body has to work to get the nutrients out of these foods, and that's good, because that gradual release helps to regulate blood sugar. Look for natural foods with more colour and fibre, since they control appetite, have more nutrients and improve your cardiovascular system.

By controlling your blood sugar, you're regulating the hormone insulin. If you're constantly pushing up your blood sugar by eating only high-glycaemic foods, crashing back down, and then eating more high-glycaemic foods, you create a vicious cycle that results in increased calorie consumption and body fat levels, obesity and perhaps even diabetes.

The reason we see so many overweight children these days, aside from an utter lack of exercise, is that much of what we feed them is high-sugar, high-glycaemic processed food that wreaks havoc on blood sugar and provides little nutritional value. Not only does this have serious health implications, it can also lead to attention deficit disorders and wild mood swings that affect development and performance throughout the day.

GLYCAEMIC INDEX OF POPULAR FOODS

LOW	MODERATE	HIGH
Apples	Bananas	Bagels
Black beans	Cheese pizza	Baked potatoes
Grapefruit	Muffins	Doughnuts
Green peas	Oat biscuits	Hamburger buns
Hummus	Pineapple	Raisins
Oranges	Porridge (not instant)	Rice cakes
Peaches	Sweetcorn	Tortilla chips

As a result, HFCS creates a vicious cycle, forcing consumers to eat more high-glycaemic food to maintain that blood sugar rush, rather than eating foods the body needs to control appetite and blood sugar level.

According to a study published in the *American Journal of Clinical Nutrition,* Americans ate an average of about 230 grams (8 ounces) of high-fructose corn syrup in 1970. By 1997, they were consuming up to 28½ kilograms (62½ pounds) each, annually! Other Western countries are catching up fast.

Ideal Players: None. Unfortunately, this sweetener is getting into everything, from soft drinks to ketchup to canned soup. It's also being added to juices, bread and every manner of processed food. Is it any wonder that obesity rates have soared over the last 3 decades?

Bottom Line: There's nothing wrong with a little high-fructose corn syrup. If it's listed first or second in the ingredients list, glance at the product's nutrition facts label to see how much sugar is in the product, and if it's more than 8 grams per serving, find a different brand or, if necessary, a healthier substitute. Generally speaking, avoid products with HFCS.

Scouting Report: Fibre
(A form of carbohydrate)

Strengths: Improves gastrointestinal health and function and helps to prevent colon cancer, regulates blood sugar and promotes long-term cardiovascular health by reducing cholesterol.

Weaknesses: None.

Ideal Players: Fibre is found in beans, many fruits, leafy green vegetables, legumes, oats, wholegrain products, as well as in supplement form. Sprinkle oat bran fibre on meals or in your shakes to improve their nutritional value.

Bottom Line: Fibre, found mostly in carbohydrates, is essential to overall health. People who follow low-carb diet plans deprive themselves of this vital source of nutrition.

Scouting Report: Proteins

Strengths: Builds, maintains and restores muscle. Responsible for ensuring we have healthy blood cells, key enzymes and strenghtening the immune system.

Weaknesses: In order to build muscle, protein must be consumed with enough carbohydrate calories to provide the body with energy. Otherwise, your body will tap into the protein for energy. Certain forms of animal proteins contain high amounts of saturated fats – for instance, heavily marbled beef.

Ideal Players:

● Fish: anchovies, calamari, cod, flounder, grouper, halibut, mackerel, monkfish, salmon, sardines, swordfish, tuna canned in water, tuna steak, sushi

● Shellfish: clams, mussels, crab, lobster, oysters, shrimp/prawns

● Poultry: chicken breast (if skinless), lean turkey mince, turkey breast

- Meat: filet mignon, flank steak, extra lean beef mince, lean ham, lean pork loin, lean steak, lean lamb steaks

- Pulses: black beans, lentils, pinto beans, refried beans (if fat-free), chick peas, kidney beans

- Dairy products: low-fat cottage cheese, egg white powder and other egg substitutes, egg whites, skimmed milk, and low-fat, low-sugar yogurt

Bottom Line: Adequate protein intake, spread throughout the day, is vital to long-term health.

I recommend that you consume 1.3 to 1.75 grams of protein per kilogram of body weight (0.6 to 0.8 grams per pound of body weight). If you weigh, say, 82 kilograms (180 pounds), you would want to shoot for between 107 and 144 grams ($3\frac{1}{2}$ to 5 ounces) of protein per day. Generally speaking, the leaner and more active you are, the higher your protein intake should be on that scale.

That might sound like a ton of protein – and it is a significant amount – but consider how much protein is in common foods such as the ones listed below.

- Chicken (115 g/4 oz, skinless, size of a pack of cards): 35 grams

- Tuna (170 g/6 oz, packed in water): 40 grams

- Fish (170 g/6 oz of cod or salmon): 40 grams

- Lean red meat (115 g/4 oz): 35 grams

- Lean pork (115 g/4 oz): 35 grams

- Reduced-fat tofu (170 g/6 oz): 30 grams

- Cottage cheese (145 g/5 oz): 28 grams

- Milk (240 ml/18 fl oz skimmed): 8 grams

Remember, too, that your pre-workout shooter or post-workout recovery mix is going to contain 20 to 45 grams ($\frac{3}{4}$ to $1\frac{1}{2}$ oz) of protein per serving. (See '"Shot Clock" Pre- and Post-Exercise Nutrition' on pages 36 to 37.) If you have one or two shakes a day, along with some combination of poultry and fish for lunch and dinner and a breakfast that includes yogurt or egg whites, you'll easily meet your daily protein goal.

In addition to 'eat a rainbow often', here's another rule of thumb regarding nutrition, specifically protein: 'the less legs, the better'. The fewer legs something has – or at least had when it was alive – the better its ratio of protein to healthy fat.

Fish, for instance, have no legs, and fish is a tremendously healthy source of protein, provided that it's not fried. Fish also provides omega-3 and omega-6 fatty acids, which promote cardiovascular health. Shellfish such as crab, lobster and prawns is the exception to 'the less legs, the better' rule. Although they have many legs, they are better for you than red meat.

Chickens have two legs and also are a wonderful source of protein, provided the skin is removed and the meat is not fried.

Meat from four-legged creatures can be good, too, provided it's a lean cut – that's a key distinction. Red meat gets bad press, some of which is deserved since the heavily marbled meats are more tender and often have more flavour. But lean red meat is a tremendous source of important nutrients such as iron and phosphorus.

Pork also gets bad press. It's usually fatty, but if you ask for a lean cut, you'll have a tasty and nutritious protein.

Scouting Report: Fats

Strengths: Critical to good health and makeup of cell membranes. Fats release energy slowly, keeping the body sated and regulating blood sugar, and thus lowering glycaemic response to other foods. Good fats provide powerful nutrients and antioxidants for cellular repair of the joints, organs, skin and hair. Fats, especially those found in fish oil and flaxseed (linseed) oil, also help with cognitive ability, mental clarity and memory retention, and they have very strong anti-inflammatory properties.

Weaknesses: Not all fat is good – and saturated fats are very bad indeed. The difference in chemical structure between saturated and unsaturated fats produces significantly different effects on health. Saturated fats, which are usually found in meat and dairy foods and are solid at room temperature, raise serum cholesterol levels, clog arteries and pose a risk to the heart.

At the same time, not all *un*saturated fats are healthy. Vegetable shortening is unsaturated, but it's unhealthy. That's because it contains trans fats, which raise bad (LDL) cholesterol but do not raise good (HDL) cholesterol. You may identify these trans fats on the label by looking for the words 'partially hydrogenated oil'. This artery-clogging fat is found in processed foods such as biscuits, crackers, pies, pastries and margarine. It's also found in fried foods, especially those at fast-food restaurants, and in smaller quantities in meat and some dairy products. As of 1 January, 2006, US food manufacturers must list on their labels the amount of trans fat; there is a drive to have similar legislation introduced in the UK. At the moment they don't have to be included on a food label unless a specific claim has been made such as 'low in trans fats'. However, many manufacturers are voluntarily putting it on the label. Look out for hydrogenated vegetable oil since it may contrain trans fats.

Ideal Players:
- Oils: fish oil, extra virgin olive oil, flaxseed (linseed) oil, rapeseed (canola) oil, soya oil

- Vegetables: avocados

- Seeds: pumpkin, sunflower, flaxseeds (linseeds)

- Nuts: almonds, cashews, pecans, macadamias, walnuts. (Almonds were found in a recent study by *Men's Health®* magazine to have the most nutritional value, followed by cashews, pecans and macadamias.)

Bottom Line: Good fats, in moderation, are great for you.

One of the biggest health trends of the last 20 years has been the anti-fat movement. Everything had to be low-fat, preferably fat-free. 'You are what you eat', according to the popular saying, and if you ate fat, you were going to end up looking like the Michelin tyre man.

The best fats come out of nuts, fish oils and seeds. Few foods have had such undeserved bad press as nuts. As part of the anti-fat movement, people avoided them because they were high in fat. But nuts and seeds are a convenient source of protein and fibre, and they stick with you longer than many snacks, helping to control blood sugar and appetite. A handful of nuts every day may lower the risk of heart ailments and Alzheimer's disease. Unsaturated fats do not raise cholesterol levels, and research indicates that they actually can reduce it when substituted for saturated fats. The best unsaturated fats, liquid at room temperature, are found in olive oil, rapeseed (canola) oil, flaxseed (linseed) oil and fish oils.

Fish oils provide powerful omega-3 and omega-6 fatty acids, which have antioxidant properties and are essential for good cardiovascular health and mental clarity. These are found in salmon, mackerel, lake trout, herring, sardines and some types of white fish. Swordfish and tuna contain fatty acids, though not as much as salmon. Fish is a tremendous source of protein, and it doesn't hit you with the unhealthy saturated fats like some fatty meats do.

Everyone should have a bottle of high-lignan flaxseed (linseed) oil and/or fish oil in the fridge. The body can convert flaxseed (linseed) oil into omega-3 and omega-6 fatty acids, much like fish oil. A tablespoon or two a day – one in the morning and one in the evening – is all you need, and it can go into a shake or on top of porridge.

Olive oil is another excellent choice. It has great antioxidant properties, is good for cooking and goes well with salads.

Scouting Report: Trans Fats

Strengths: None, though food manufacturers love the fact that it's so cheap and easy to create trans fat by adding hydrogen to vegetable oil – a process called hydrogenation. Hydrogenation increases the shelf life and flavour of the foods containing these fats.

Weaknesses: Trans fat raises the LDL cholesterol that increases the risk of heart disease. According to a 9-year study of 16,500 men published in the *American Journal of Clinical Nutrition,* researchers found that for every 2 per cent increase in trans fat intake, men added one-third of an inch to their waists over the course of a year.

Ideal Players: None. Trans fat is found everywhere – in vegetable shortenings, some margarines, biscuits, crackers, snack foods and other foods made with or fried in partially hydrogenated oils.

Bottom Line: Try to avoid all products that contain trans fat.

CORE NUTRITION STRATEGY 4: STAY HYDRATED

We tend to take water for granted. It's readily available, but instead we hydrate with inferior drinks ranging from fizzy drinks to coffee to alcohol. For all of the advances in technology, we still have not come up with something better than water. It's the perfect drink.

If I said that you could do up to 25 per cent more work or run 25 per cent further, you'd sprint through a wall to make that happen, wouldn't you? Actually, it's much easier. Just drink enough water before, during and after exercise. Drink 4.5 litres (1 gallon) of water a day. Drink 480 ml (16 fl oz) of water first thing in the morning. Take a couple of 1.5-litre (2½-pint) bottles to work and drink all day. Keep a bottle in the car.

If you want to reduce calories quickly, cut them out of your drinks. If you replace soft drinks, juices, sports drinks and beer with water, you'll cut down on calories and sugar. Without those calories for energy, your body will burn body fat and the higher-fibre carbs recommended by the Core Nutrition game plan for energy. You'll lose fat and probably weight, too. For convenience, buy a pack of bottled water and keep the bottles nearby in the fridge. That way you're more likely to grab water instead of other sugary drinks.

Water has a direct impact on the ageing process. Because of dehydration, inactivity and trauma from daily life, the connective tissues around our muscles and joints dry up over time, sort of like those chew toys for dogs that start out soft and pliable and end up stiff and brittle after a lot of chewing. Drinking lots of water slows this process while improving your muscle tissue and flexibility.

As far as artificial sweeteners in soft drinks and other beverages go, recent research suggests that *modest* consumption of artificial sweeteners is a better alternative to high-fructose corn syrup and other sugars. Although I'm not a fan of diet soft drinks – it is better to drink water – they are a much better choice than a regular soft drink that's loaded with sugar. (A typical can of 'regular' soft drink has about 150 calories, all from sugar.)

Instead of drinking caffeine-filled coffee, consider a healthier alternative such as green, white or black tea. All of these teas have protective antioxidant properties.

Proper hydration regulates appetite. Often, people think they're hungry when they're really just thirsty. If you're trying to lose weight, have a glass of water before eating – it will help to prevent you from overeating.

Always 'think before you drink'. Are you drinking to stay hydrated, or to produce a certain response? If you substitute water for coffee, fizzy drinks and alcohol, you'll have no problem drinking 4.5 litres (1 gallon) a day. Drink two glasses when you wake up, two glasses with every meal, and plenty of water before, during and after working out. You won't miss the caffeine. The Core Nutrition game plan will help you to regulate your blood sugar and maintain your energy level, so you won't feel quite the need to use caffeine as an artificial energy source.

Don't assume that sports drinks are an adequate substitute for water, especially in everyday life. In fact, most are loaded with a ton of high-glycaemic carbohydrates that elevate blood sugar and ultimately contribute to body fat (though sports drinks are critical for serious endurance athletes and for other athletes who compete in prolonged, intense activity). One of the most exciting hydration products to hit the market is made by one of my company's sponsors, Amino Vital, which contains a combination of branched chain amino acids (BCAAs), arginine and glutamine to support immune health, muscle recovery and improve mental function.

Scouting Report: Wine

Strengths: Studies suggest that moderate consumption of red wine reduces the risk of cardiovascular disease. Resveratrol, an antioxidant, is found in high concentrations in red grape skins. Some people also find that red wine enhances their enjoyment of food, especially red meats.

Weaknesses: Besides the obvious dangers of excessive alcohol consumption, alcohol also impairs our deep REM (rapid eye movement) sleep, which is essential for positive hormone release, body repair and quality sleep. Alcohol consists of empty calories and lessens immune function. It decreases performance, slows the recovery process, impairs judgement, causes dehydration and, of course, is addictive.

Ideal Players: Pinot Noir, Beaujolais, Shiraz, Merlot, Cabernet Sauvignon. If you don't drink alcohol, consider adding grape juice or grape seed extract supplements to your diet, to obtain antioxidant properties similar to those found in resveratrol.

Bottom Line: Alcohol contains 7 empty calories per gram and should be consumed only in moderation. One glass of red wine, a few times per week, is an acceptable part of the Core Nutrition programme. Always consume one glass of water for each alcoholic drink to prevent dehydration.

Chapter 4 Summary: A few simple nutritional strategies will make a dramatic impact on your health. Eat smaller portions more often, spread evenly across the day, containing a combination of lean protein, healthy fats and less-processed carbohydrates. Your carbohydrate intake should be relative to your activity level. Eat 'glycaemically correct' carbs, high in colour and fibre – the less processed, the better. Drink plenty of water, and add a pre-workout shooter or post-workout recovery mix to your routine.

CHAPTER 5

GAME PLAN

I n order to eat properly, you need to forget the traditional concept of the word *diet.* The connotation is negative – the first three letters are d-i-e – and diets are viewed as quick-fix, temporary solutions. From this point forwards, you will have to make a conscious decision every time you eat something. Turn off your bad-habit autopilot and ask yourself, 'Will this help me achieve my goals, or sabotage them?'

Start viewing your nutrition programme as a game plan for your long-term health and productivity. It's a vital, core strategy for the rest of your life. Otherwise you take a reactive approach to eating, consuming whatever is out there, with little thought to how it affects you, in terms of both energy production and long-term health.

As with everything else in this book, I want you to be proactive about your diet. I recommend that you take 90 minutes each Saturday or Sunday to plan, shop and prepare menus of meals for an entire week. It's easy and fun – and it saves money and time.

The problem with many diet plans is that they make you go cold turkey. *We're* not going to do that. Instead, let's take a more realistic approach.

CREATING THE
HOME GROUND ADVANTAGE

Let's start in your kitchen. Think of yourself as the general manager of a sports team. In pro

CORE NUTRITION: 3 WEEKS TO RESHAPE YOUR LIFE

Week One: 'Training Camp, 4 on 4'

We're going to stock the cupboards, fridge and freezer properly. We're going to eat four meals a day – 4 days a week. The other 3 days? Try to do the same, but don't worry if you don't quite make it.

Week Two: 'Pre-season, 5 on 5'

Now we're going to eat five meals a day – 5 days a week. Again, don't worry about the other 2 days.

Week Three: 'Regular Season (and beyond), 6 on 6'

We're going to eat six meals a day, 6 days a week. Use the other day to eat what you like.

sports, the 'GM' must work within constraints. He has a set budget. Perhaps there's some dead weight on the roster in the form of long-term, guaranteed contracts of players now injured or ineffective. No matter how hard the GM tries, he cannot dump those contracts on someone else.

Many people approach the assembly of their kitchen cupboards and fridges the same way, even though they're not bound by any constraints. There's plenty of dead weight – both the junk in the cupboards and the fat it has heaped on their bodies – but still, people continue to purchase more unhealthy food. They're like general managers that keep acquiring underachieving, expensive players that keep the team from winning.

If you look inside your cupboards and fridge and see foods with little nutritional value, chances are you're not going to like what you see in the mirror either. How we look is a direct reflection of how we fuel our bodies and the amount of physical activity we engage in.

Embarking on a new nutrition programme is impossible if your kitchen is filled with temptation. In order to eat properly, you must control the environment. I cannot stress enough how much our environment supports our habits, especially at home. It's more challenging to eat right when out of the house, especially while travelling. So at least give yourself a home ground advantage by stocking your kitchen properly. If there's nothing bad in the house to eat, chances are you're going to eat properly.

We're going to 'draft' a new team of good foods. But first, let's cut all of those bad players from our roster. Unlike the general manager, we're not stuck with anything. Take a garbage bin and go into the kitchen. Toss away all those processed foods, such as biscuits, crackers, crisps, white pastas and rice, cake mixes, sweets, creamy soups, sugary cereals and fizzy drinks. Open the fridge and discard beer, whole milk, creamy side dishes and casseroles, ice cream, fatty meats, white bread – anything that's not a high-performance food.

Wow, look at all that space you have! Now it's time to go to the supermarket and draft a new team of players. Don't worry if you don't know where to find them, even if you've been shopping in the same place for years. We tend to be creatures of habit, rolling down the aisles on autopilot, grabbing the same foods we've eaten forever. But if you take just a moment and consider some healthier alternatives, many of which taste better, you can change your life. You'll look and feel better, have more energy and live longer.

As you look inside that empty kitchen, you might wonder if there are any foods left out there. In fact, there are dozens. On page 50 is a list of foods we're going to obtain. I recommend that you photocopy the list and keep it in your wallet or handbag, or even in the glove compartment of your car.

THE DRAFT: LET'S GO SHOPPING

Now that you have your Core Nutrition strategies in place, we are going to arm you with a Core Nutrition shopping list and a map of the Core supermarket for recruiting the right players.

Before we go, it's important for you to understand how to get around the ground – and manage to stay in bounds. We also have provided complete scouting reports for each department and the right shopping aisles. Fuel up before you go; it's never a good idea to shop hungry.

As you work through the supermarket, stay along the perimeter. Virtually everything you need is along the outer aisles, such as produce, fish, meat and dairy products. Instead of going down every aisle, glance at the overhead signs to locate healthy items such as tinned tuna fish, beans, frozen fruits, vegetables, protein, porridge oats and olive oil. Leave the trolley at one end and walk down the aisle. That way you avoid being tempted by cake mixes, biscuits, crisps and soft drinks. And you'll save time, too.

Most of us learn about foods from the worst possible places – the media, and, more specifically, advertisers. Much of what we hear from these sources isn't accurate, and what is accurate is at best incomplete. You have to fill in the blanks. Examine labels for content, especially the amounts of proteins, fats and carbs contained. If you're good with numbers, try to calculate the percentages of each in the food. Look at the line that tells you how many grams of sugar are in the product, then look at the list of ingredients to see what kind of sugar it is. I've already explained that high-fructose corn syrup (or HFCS) is to be avoided. The same goes for trans fats.

All this reading and calculating might take a few extra minutes at first, but pretty soon you'll be able to cruise through the aisles – maybe even faster than before.

Though I use the term *supermarket,* I recognize that some people shop at independent retailers or large discount supermarkets. Buying bigger sizes of Core Nutrition staples will save

(continued on page 52)

CORE GROCERY LIST

GENERAL SHOPPING TIPS:

● Stay focused. ● Avoid products displayed at the heads of the aisles.
● Watch out at the checkout! ● Explore one new healthy food with each shopping trip.

BAKERY
100% wholemeal bread
Wholegrain bread

CEREAL AISLE
Bran cereal
Kashi cereal (my personal favourite)
Porridge oats

TINNED FOODS
Black beans
Chick peas
Fruit, packaged with no sugar added
Kidney beans
Haricot beans
Pinto beans
Tuna, water-packed

DELI SECTION
TIP: Avoid deli salads and fried foods.
Deli meats, lean and reduced-fat
Hummus
Rotisserie chicken (remove skin and pat down chicken)

MEAT & SEAFOOD AISLES
Chicken, skinless, white meat
Minced beef, extra lean
Red meat and pork, lean
Salmon and other fish
Turkey, white meat

DAIRY SECTION
TIP: Avoid full-cream milk products.
Cheese, low-fat
Cottage cheese

Juices, 100% juice, no sugar added
Milk, skimmed
Tofu
Yogurt, low-fat, low-sugar

FROZEN FOODS
Fruits
Ice cream, low-fat, low-sugar
Juices, 100% juice, no sugar added
Soya yogurt
Vegetables

BAKING, SNACK AND CONDIMENT AISLES
Almonds
Flaxseed (linseed) oil
High-protein meal-replacement bars
Mustard
Olive oil
Peanut butter, natural
Peanuts
Rapeseed (Canola) oil
Salad dressing, low-fat
Soya oil
Sunflower seeds
Vinegar, balsamic or red wine (for salads)

FRUIT AND VEGETABLE SECTION
TIPS: Stock it up!
Cut and package produce to eat later.
Apples, red or green
Apricots

Bananas
Blueberries
Broccoli
Carrots
Cauliflower
Cucumber
Grapefruit
Grapes, red
Green beans
Kiwi fruit
Oranges
Pears
Romaine lettuce
Spinach
Strawberries
Sweet potatoes
Tomatoes

PHARMACY
Antioxidant complex
Calcium (for women)
Fish oil/omega-3 capsules
Multivitamin
Vitamin C (500 mg)
Vitamin E (400 IU)
Whey protein powder

DRINKS AISLES
Coffee, regular and decaf
Herbal Tea, such as Peppermint or Camomile
Juices, 100% juice, no sugar added
Tea, green, white and black
Water, bottled
Wine, red

SERVING SIZES
Vegetables: 185 g/6½ oz raw vegetables, 90 g/3 oz cooked vegetables, 150 ml/¼ pt vegetable juice, 170 g/6 oz cooked dry beans
Fruits: 1 medium-size fruit (1 medium apple or 1 medium pear), 150 g/5½ oz canned or chopped fruit, or 150 ml/¼ pt fruit juice
Breads and Cereals: 1 slice of bread, 40 g/1¼ oz ready-to-eat cereal, 170 g/6 oz cooked rice or pasta
Protein: 115 g/4 oz meat (the size of the palm of your hand), handful of nuts, 2 tbsp peanut butter
Fats: 1 tbsp olive oil, 1 tbsp rapeseed (canola) oil, 1 tbsp flaxseed (linseed) oil, 1 tbsp fish oil
Dairy: 240 ml/8 fl oz milk, 150 g/5½ oz cottage cheese, 30 g/1 oz or slice of cheese

CORE SUPERMARKET DIAGRAM

Stay along the perimeter of the store. Avoid the middle aisles, except for the occasional healthy item.

you money. You'll also save time since you can freeze what you don't use.

Now, let's go aisle by aisle through the supermarket and fill your shopping trolley with high-quality Core foods. We've provided a scouting report for each area. Now it's time to go shopping.

Scouting Report: Dairy

Strengths: Dairy products are good sources of calcium, which supports bones. New research suggests that calcium intake may help to lower body fat.

Weaknesses: Dairy products can add unnecessary calories to a meal. They often can be high in fat.

Ideal/Undervalued Players: Skimmed milk; low-fat cottage cheese and cream cheese; fat-free or low-fat natural yogurt.

Pretenders: Low-fat and fat-free flavoured yogurt often is loaded with empty calories in the form of sugar, which will send your blood sugar level soaring.

Bottom Line: Dairy products, in moderation, are good sources of calcium.

Scouting Report: Fruits and Vegetables

Strengths: It's hard to go wrong in this section of the store. Since you want to 'eat a rainbow often', you should fill up a good chunk of your trolley right here. Fruit and vegetable platters are healthy alternatives to crisps and dips to serve at parties. Prepackaged salads often can be found in the deli section. Garden salads are fine, provided

that the dressing is on the side. Go easy on the croutons. As always, the more colour, the better. Salads with leafy spinach and romaine lettuce tend to be more colourful and nutrient-dense than those made predominantly with iceberg lettuce.

Weaknesses: None. This is the healthiest part of the supermarket.

Ideal Players: Foods rich in colour and anti-oxidant properties, such as tomatoes, blueberries, spinach, asparagus, pomegranates and broccoli. Salads with plenty of spinach and tomatoes are also terrific.

Undervalued Prospects: Just about any colourful, fibre-rich vegetable is undervalued. Soyabeans are another power food. They're rich in nutrients and high in protein.

Pretenders: Dried fruit and nut mixes. They're calorie-dense and too heavy in sugar. Iceberg lettuce has little nutritional value.

Bottom Line: When choosing fruits and vegetables, fresh is the best way to go. Frozen fruit and veggies are preferable to tinned goods, since nutrients are lost in the canning process.

Scouting Report: Deli

Strengths: Lean meat is a rich and convenient source of protein.

Weaknesses: Cheese is tempting for many people. When you eat cheese, do so in moderation – ideally, treat it as a garnish.

Ideal Players: Less than 5 per cent fat (5 g fat per 100 g) deli-sliced meats, and low-fat deli-sliced cheeses (in moderation). Generally speaking, softer cheeses have lower fat content, whereas hard cheese usually contains more of the unhealthy saturated fats. Eat cheese only in moderation.

Undervalued Prospects: Rotisserie chicken is one of my favourites. It's flavourful, it's pre-cooked and it provides several meals out of a single chicken at an affordable price. The key is to drain the fat, remove the fatty skin and pat the bird down with a paper towel.

Pretenders: Pasta salads, potato salad and other creamy side dishes.

Bottom Line: You always want to go for the leanest cuts of meat and cheese possible. When selecting turkey, ham and chicken, go for products that contain less than 5 per cent fat.

Scouting Report: Bread and Baked Goods

Strengths: This is an area where we may find some great low-glycaemic, high-fibre carbohydrates.

Weaknesses: Avoid white and buttermilk refined breads; they have too much refined flour. Be on the lookout for high-fructose corn syrup; it even appears in bread. Bagels and teacakes should be eaten only in the morning and with the proper toppings (natural peanut butter, reduced-fat cheese spread such as Philadelphia Light). As for tortillas, go for the wholewheat, low-carb version where possible.

Ideal Players: Tough to draft an ideal player here. If you eat bread, look for 'stone-ground'. Wholemeal breads marketed as 'light' generally tend to come in thinner slices, which is another way to keep from overdoing it on breads.

Undervalued Prospects: Wholegrain breads, such as rye and pumpernickel, typically fall in a lower range on the glycaemic index than wholemeal bread. This can be an advantage in controlling blood sugar and energy. Wholemeal, however, can have more fibre than the other breads. Judging solely by glycaemic rating, a wholegrain bread might be superior, but because of its fibre content, wholemeal bread is the winner in this section.

Pretenders: White breads, along with cake mixes, muffins and brownies – pretty much the entire baked goods aisle.

Bottom Line: When choosing breads, opt for wholegrain or wholemeal, which have not been heavily processed. Don't be fooled by loaves of brown bread labelled as 'wheat'. If it's not made with wholemeal flour, it's just white bread dyed to look like something more nutritious.

Scouting Report: Condiments, Jams and Spices

Strengths: Condiments don't add much nutritional value but small quantities make food tasty, ensuring that you'll stay with the programme.

Weaknesses: Condiment labelling can be deceiving. Salad dressings are notoriously confusing. One manufacturer's 'low-fat' might be comparable to the standard brand of another company. Whatever you choose, go easy on the dressing. It also pays to read the jam labels. The lower the sugar content, the better. Straight fruit spreads (as opposed to preserves) are preferable.

Ideal Players: Hummus is an exotic blend of lemon, chickpeas, garlic, sesame puree and olive oil that contains no saturated fat, cholesterol or sugar. It also contains protein and fibre. Spices such as oregano and parsley are a great way to add flavour to your food without adding lots of calories.

Replace butter with a lower-calorie substitute such as a soft low-fat spread (be sure to check there are no trans fats in it). Sprays are preferable to tub margarines, since most people have a tendency to go overboard with spreads. You get better coverage and use less if you choose a spray. Olive oil or 'Fry Light' oils are ideal for cooking.

Undervalued Prospects: Mustard, hummus, salsa and horseradish are better alternatives to mayonnaise. Olive oil and balsamic vinegar are preferable to salad dressing. Extra virgin olive oil is best; it's produced from the first pressing of olives and has less than 1 per cent acidity.

Peanut butter gets a bad press. *Natural* peanut butter is better than run-of-the-mill creamy brands. Pour off about half of the oil floating at the top of natural peanut butter, and mix up the rest. If you must go with a standard peanut butter, be careful with the low-fat products. Manufacturers tend to pour in the high-fructose corn syrup.

Replace sugar with Splenda, a no-calorie sweetener that is made, according to its Web site, 'through a patented process that starts with sugar and converts it to a no-calorie, non-carbohydrate sweetener'.

Pretenders: Sugar, butter, mayonnaise, anything with high-fructose corn syrup.

Bottom Line: Spend some time reading the labels in this aisle. Whether it's salad dressing, barbecue sauce, ketchup or mayonnaise, it's important to examine the grams of fat and sugar and the number of calories per serving.

Scouting Report: Cereals and Breakfast Foods

Strengths: With breakfast being the most important meal of the day, this aisle provides the quickest and easiest options.

Weaknesses: Besides being ridiculously expensive, many cereals provide only modest nutritional value. Too often, they're loaded with sugar and calories.

Ideal Players: Good old fashioned porridge oats have been around forever but are still arguably the best cereal option. The 1-minute version and low-sugar prepackaged oatmeal products are more processed, but they still make a decent choice. The original Cheerios also are a good choice since they, too, are made from oats. Avoid the sugary versions of Cheerios. Lean breakfast meats and low-fat, low-sugar yogurts are also great choices.

Undervalued Prospects: Kashi's breakfast cereals are high in fibre and full of nutrients. They make an excellent breakfast choice. Egg whites or similar substitutes are preferable to eggs. For those times when you do bake, consider replacing whole eggs partially or fully with egg whites. (Two egg whites are equivalent to one egg.) Again, make the best choice possible, even if you're eating cake.

Pretenders: Sugary cereals, French toast, doughnuts, pastries, most waffles and pancakes, sugary fruit drinks.

Bottom Line: It's important to get the day started right. Rethink that big breakfast. For instance, pancakes are permissible as long as you don't make a complete meal out of them. There's nothing wrong with having one pancake with, say, an egg-white omelette. Use low fat, trans fat free spread instead of butter on your pancake. Use syrup sparingly and look for brands with little or no sugar.

Scouting Report: Fish and Meat

Strengths: Fish and meat are tremendous sources of protein, the building blocks of muscle.

Weaknesses: Some cuts of meat tend to be heavily marbled with those dangerous saturated animal fats.

Ideal Players: Salmon is one of the best power foods. Besides being a better source of protein than most meats, it's loaded with omega-3 fatty acids, which have heart disease–reducing properties. Not only that, but many people also find salmon more flavourful than other fish.

Undervalued Prospects: Contrary to popular belief, lean red meat is great for you. Lean cuts are high in protein, low in fat and great sources of iron and phosphorus. Red meat should be consumed in moderation, but there's no reason to eliminate it from your diet.

A good strategy is to select cuts made from the animal's muscles of locomotion. Lean steaks come from the rear legs. Flank cuts also are very lean and so is cubed steak. Avoid fattier, more marbled cuts such as strips, stewing steak and T-bones. Lean pork is also a terrific choice, especially when grilled.

Tinned tuna fish is an excellent source of protein; just make sure it's tinned in water, not vegetable oil.

Pretenders: Fatty meat, battered or breaded fish, creamy seafood salads.

Bottom Line: Remember the rule: the less legs, the better. It's tough to go wrong with fish, though it should be baked or grilled – never fried or breaded. After fish, chicken and other types of poultry have the fewest legs. Game birds are a good alternative, though like chicken they should be stripped of skin. As with fish, poultry never should be fried or breaded.

Scouting Report: Pasta and Side Dishes

Strengths: Not many. A small, tennis-ball-size serving of pasta – preferably wholewheat or vegetable pasta – is acceptable. Go with low-sugar, meatless pasta sauce. Add lycopene-rich tomato purée and a little olive oil, or make your own sauce, adding extra-lean minced beef or turkey and herbs for flavour.

Weaknesses: Pasta is high-glycaemic, and it has a very high glycaemic load, meaning that a small portion can send blood sugar levels soaring very quickly.

Ideal Players: Wholewheat pasta in small quantities. When choosing rice, go with brown rice, wild rice and basmati rice rather than white rice. Brown rice has more fibre than white rice, because it's less processed.

Undervalued Prospects: A better alternative to rice is couscous. Pronounced 'koos-koos,' it's a staple of North African cooking and is made from durum wheat, the ideal pasta wheat because of its high protein content.

Pretenders: Overcooked pastas, white pastas, white rice.

Bottom Line: The key to pasta and rice is to go whole grain, don't cook them very long and look at them as a side dish, not as an entire meal.

Scouting Report: Snacks

Strengths: Low-glycaemic, nutrient-dense snacks are a quick and easy way to control mid-afternoon hunger pangs.

Weaknesses: If you have a hankering for something sweet, try a low-sugar frozen-fruit bar or a reduced fat ice lolly. When choosing ice cream or frozen yogurt, look for brands that are low in fat and sugar. Buy small containers of ice cream, since studies suggest that the larger the container, the larger the serving a person will take.

Ideal Players: Almonds; sunflower seeds; low-fat yogurt with no sugar added (add in fibre with oats, nuts, seeds or a teaspoon of flaxseed/linseed or fish oil); fruits; veggies; good protein snack bars (see below).

Undervalued Prospects: Protein bars can be a great late-afternoon 'meal'. Unfortunately, many of these so-called meal-replacement bars have the same nutritional value as chocolate bars. Ideally, look for a snack bar that has a carbs-to-protein ratio of no more than 2:1 – generally, the more protein, the better. So if a bar has 30 grams (1 ounce) of carbs, it should have at least 15 grams (½ ounce) of protein. Many products have a higher ratio of protein, such as 1:2, meaning 15 grams (½ ounce) of carbs and 30 grams (1 ounce) of protein.

Pretenders: Granola bars, cereal bars, dried fruit, high-sugar yogurts, all other sugary products, salted and sugary nuts, and high-fat, low nutrient-value crackers, etc. This last option tends to be highly processed, calorie-dense and high in sugar and/or bad fats.

Bottom Line: Individual preferences vary widely when it comes to meal-replacement bars. If you've had bad experiences with them in the past, give them another chance.

Scouting Report: Drinks

Strengths: Proper hydration is essential for health.

Weaknesses: For many people, life is impossible without coffee. The Core Performance Essentials programme, which emphasizes proper sleep and meal timing, should help to wean you away from your caffeine addiction.

When you do drink coffee, don't order a 'grande', and don't overdo the cream and sugar. Try Splenda instead of sugar, and skimmed milk rather than full cream.

If you must have soft drinks, go with a diet version. I don't advocate diet soft drinks by any means – giving up soft drinks might be the easiest way for you to get more water – but if you must have them, find a diet brand you like. These will keep you hydrated, but water still is the best choice.

Ideal Players: Water is *the* ideal drink. Pick up a case of 500 ml or 1.5-litre bottles to take to work, to the gym or to keep in your car when you're out running errands. If you live in an area with poor-quality water, buy a water filter, or use a water distiller or filtration jug.

Undervalued Prospects: Green or white tea is a great substitute for coffee. I call them 'power drinks', since they're natural sources of antioxidants. If you must have sugar with your coffee or tea, go with Splenda. Skimmed milk is better than whole or semi-skimmed. This rule applies to all dairy products.

Be careful when choosing fruit juices or fruit drinks – they often have too much sugar and high-fructose corn syrup. Always look for alternatives that are 100 per cent fruit juice. Most juice can be diluted further with water, which lowers its glycaemic load. You'll also get more

out of it, which is a good thing since juice, like cereal, is usually overpriced.

Pretenders: Fizzy and fruit drinks. Choose sports drinks for the right reason – to help you train for endurance sports; make sure they don't contain high-fructose corn syrup, a standard ingredient in many sport and fruit drinks.

Bottom Line: Unless you're a serious endurance athlete or doing a lot of strength training, someone who's involved in running, cycling or other strenuous activities for long periods of time, you probably don't need anything more than water. You definitely don't need sports drinks for routine refreshment around the house or at work. (Remember: think before you drink. Avoid drinking empty calories.)

Chapter 5 Summary: We have prepared ourselves for success by rewiring our mindset and creating powerful changes in our environment. Unlike traditional, quick-fix diet plans, the Core Nutrition programme is a long-term plan to fuel your body for maximum daily energy and long-term success. Instead of requiring you to go cold turkey, this programme includes a 3-week indoctrination programme. Each meal should consist of a lean protein source along with low- to mid-glycaemic, colourful and fibre-rich carbohydrates, and healthy fats in moderation. Always strive to make the best choice possible.

WINNING AT HOME

Planning is the key to eating properly, and over the next 3 weeks you're going to change the way you eat. In Week One, we'll do away with all of those bad foods and start eating four quality meals a day, 4 days a week. We'll stock our kitchen and office, as we will discuss in this chapter. In Week Two, we'll build upon that momentum and go for five good meals a day, 5 days a week.

Now that we have these empowering foods around, it's tough to make a bad decision. Not only that, but we also feel great about the decisions we're making because we can see the benefit of all this effort. We're starting to transform our bodies and are producing more energy. We're starting to benefit from these new routines.

By Week Three, we will have established habits for life. We have the energy and a plan to sustain it regardless of what gets thrown at us in the Game of Life.

If you fail nutritionally, it's almost certainly due to a lack of planning. So, instead of embarking on a mere diet, we're going to make a lifestyle change to produce more energy and protect the immune system. This will be the foundation for everything we do. We now have home ground advantage.

You don't have to be perfect all the time.

Remember, you're approaching this like an athlete, and even the best athletes do not create perfect results. A great football player might not score a goal in every game. The best tennis players sometimes serve double faults. From time to time, you will fall off this plan, and that's okay. But just jump right back on; you only fail if you give up.

One of the key components to my work with professional athletes is what I call 'motivation through education'. I could just tell you to consume the foods listed above and hope you'll follow my suggestions. But you'll be much more motivated once you understand *why* we're eating this way, and you'll know that you can pull it off because we have given you the simple strategies you need for success.

Eating well, like working out properly, is a matter of understanding a few concepts, which we have shared with you, and creating a great plan to implement them. If you have the proper nutrition system in place, you'll find that eating healthily is less stressful, less expensive and more enjoyable.

I'll show you how to get the most nutrients out of your foods and how to create a champi-

SUNDAY – THE 'OFF' DAY

Schedule one day a week that you call your 'off' day from training and nutrition. Since Sunday is an off day from the Core Workout, feel free to take the day off nutritionally as well. This doesn't mean that you should consume an entire lasagne with a six-pack and a slice of chocolate gateau, but it's okay to treat yourself. You've worked hard all week and you deserve to relax. Not only that, but having that treat provides a psychological benefit: it helps you to realize that you're not completely depriving yourself of foods you enjoy, even if they aren't particularly good for you.

It's unrealistic to think that you're going to eat nothing but healthy foods. So take Sundays off. Remember, even elite pros who train at Athletes' Performance allow themselves an occasional indulgence.

Don't be surprised, however, if many of those foods you used to love no longer seem appealing. You'll find that they no longer make you feel good, even in the short term. Once you've made this connection, feeling the response from your body, that's when you know you've taken this programme to a higher level.

Sunday should also be your day to plan the week ahead. Shop, prepare meals and create a game plan for the coming week's meals and snacks. Use Sunday to pat yourself on the back for the successful regeneration.

onship meal plan that includes the proper amount of proteins, carbs, fats, fibre, vitamins and minerals. You'll see how to combine foods into tasty meals that have a powerful nutritional value and to maximize energy.

CORE MEAL 1:
MAKE BREAKFAST THE MOST IMPORTANT MEAL OF THE DAY

Think of breakfast as 'break-the-fast', which is exactly what you're doing. When you wake up in the morning, your body is in a fasted state. During sleep, it uses the available nutrients for repair and energy, and by the time you wake up, there's usually nothing left. Your tank is empty, and the body will turn to your lean muscle stores for energy.

By skipping breakfast, as many people do, you actually increase the risk of obesity. In fact, researchers at the University of Massachusetts in the US found that not eating breakfast increases the risk of obesity by 450 per cent! Eating breakfast *away* from home increased the risk 137 per cent, no doubt because you're less likely to eat immediately and less likely to eat healthily.

Since we'll have a nutrient-dense, slow-releasing snack before bedtime, we're going to give the body what it wants so that it doesn't tap into its lean muscle stores. Breakfast is going to ensure that your body doesn't consume its muscle for food, a process known as *catabolism.* Breakfast also increases metabolism, fuels the brain and provides energy.

It's important that breakfast include protein, fibre-rich carbohydrates *and* good fats. You can add a small glass of 100 per cent fruit juice or a larger glass of diluted 100 per cent fruit juice to make a complete breakfast. The key here is buying 100 per cent fruit juice, which is quite different to a 'fruit drink' with real juice added. These fruit drinks are usually sweetened with high-fructose corn syrup and don't have the nutritional value of real juice.

Instead of drinking juice, why not try eating the original fruit with a glass of water? Consume an orange instead of juice. There's nothing wrong with OJ, of course, but remember that because it's already been processed for you, it's going to give you a higher glycaemic response than the piece of fruit itself. Eating an orange also gives you added fibre and nutrients. Let your body be the manufacturing plant, squeezing out all the nutrients that the orange has to offer.

Another good option is low-fat, low-sugar yogurt, which tastes great, sticks with you longer than the sugary types and helps to regulate blood sugar levels. It also can be a good source of protein and digestive enzymes. Add in some extra fibre, nuts or flaxseeds (linseeds). It's also tasty mixed with porridge.

Top Power Breakfasts

'Breakfast Goulash'

40 g/1¼ oz uncooked oats

1½ scoops whey protein powder

60 ml/2 fl oz water

170 g/6 oz low-fat, low-sugar yogurt

10 almonds

1 teaspoon flaxseed (linseed) oil

Stir the oats and whey protein powder together dry. Add the water and stir wet. Add the yogurt, almonds and flaxseed (linseed) oil. Enjoy!

Makes 1 serving.

RECIPE NUTRIENT ANALYSIS (PER SERVING)
503 Calories (kcal), 20 g Protein, 60 g Carbohydrates, 20 g Fat, 12.5g Saturated Fat, 4g Total Dietary Fibre

'Hot Stuff'

1 packet porridge oats

160 ml/6 fl oz water

170 g/6 oz low-fat/low-sugar yogurt or unsweetened applesauce

3 capsules fish oil

Heat the oats and water for 2 minutes. Add the yogurt or applesauce and the fish oil capsules. (Don't break the capsules open.) Serve with a bottle of water.

Makes 1 serving.

RECIPE NUTRIENT ANALYSIS (PER SERVING)
(YOGURT VERSION)
247 Calories (kcal), 12 g Protein, 36 g Carbohydrates, 7 g Fat, 1 g Saturated Fat, 3 g Total Dietary Fibre

RECIPE NUTRIENT ANALYSIS (PER SERVING)
(APPLESAUCE VERSION)
231 Calories (kcal), 4 g Protein, 40 g Carbohydrates, 6 g Fat, 1 g Saturated Fat, 4 g Total Dietary Fibre

Breakfast Bagel

1 egg

1 egg white

1 slice lean back bacon

1 slice low-fat Cheddar cheese

1 wholemeal bagel

In a small bowl, whisk the egg and egg white together. Pour into a microwave-safe bowl that is about the size of a bagel, and microwave on high power for 60 to 70 seconds. Top the egg mixture with the bacon and cheese. Microwave for another 50 to 60 seconds. Meanwhile, slice the bagel in half and toast it. Turn the egg mixture onto 1 bagel half, and top with the other half.

Makes 1 serving.

RECIPE NUTRIENT ANALYSIS (PER SERVING)
376 Calories (kcal), 30 g Protein, 34 g Carbohydrates, 14 g Fat, 5 g Saturated Fat, 4 g Total Dietary Fibre

CORE MEALS 2 AND 3: FOR LUNCH AND DINNER, THINK COMBO

When planning lunch and dinner, it's vital to include a combination of lean protein and some brightly coloured carbs that are rich in fibre. You want to have some good fat, too, from olive oil, fish, nuts or seeds. The foods will balance each other to produce maximum energy, build lean mass and regulate your blood sugar level.

We have a tendency in our busy culture to skip lunch or eat something on the run that offers poor nutritional value, but you should take the time to pack your lunch the night before. Always take a designated time to eat lunch and relax for a few minutes, even if you get stuck in the office. Sit down and eat lunch away from your desk if possible. It helps to break up the day and refreshed you for a more productive afternoon. Don't wait until you are starving to eat. Be more proactive and control your hunger; don't let it control you.

When planning dinners, consider everyone's schedules; it's important information that will help you plan accordingly. Are you preparing dinner for one, two or more. Do you need to prepare enough for everyone and set some aside for when they actually arrive? Good scheduling will also help you to block out time to get everyone around one table, so that you can nourish your personal relationships while you are nourishing your body.

Top Power Assemblies for Lunch or Dinner

Surprisingly Simple Salmon

1 tbsp olive oil

Fish seasoning to taste

1 145-g/5-oz salmon fillet

1 285-g/10-oz bag of fresh baby spinach, prewashed

15 baby tomatoes

Add the olive oil to a medium pan and heat on medium-high. Sprinkle the seasoning on both sides of the salmon and add the salmon to the pan. Pan-sear for 3 to 6 minutes on each side. Add the spinach and tomatoes. Cover and cook for 2 minutes, or until the fish is opaque and the spinach is wilted. Take the salmon out of the pan and pat it with a paper towel. Put the salmon in the centre of a plate and surround it with the cooked vegetables.

Makes 1 serving.

RECIPE NUTRIENT ANALYSIS (PER SERVING)
480 Calories (kcal), 37 g Protein, 11 g Carbohydrates, 30 g Fat, 5 g Saturated Fat, 8 g Total Dietary Fibre

BBQ Salmon

2 115-g/4-oz salmon fillets

6 tbsp low-fat dressing

Salt and ground black pepper to taste

45 g/1½ oz low-fat Cheddar cheese

1 wholemeal pita

Heat the grill to medium-high. Coat the shiny side of a large piece of aluminium foil with cooking spray. Place it shiny side up on the grill rack.

Place the salmon fillets on the foil and coat each one with 3 tablespoons of the dressing. Sprinkle the top of each fillet with salt and pepper, then fold the foil up only around the edges so that the fish simmers in its own juice while exposed.

Continue grilling the salmon for 12 to 20 minutes, or until white bubbles appear on the top of the salmon. (It should be flaky when done.) Remove the fish from the grill and serve.

It's delicious with steamed, frozen organic broccoli sprinkled with low-fat grated cheese; tomato slices; and pita bread.

Makes 2 servings.

RECIPE NUTRIENT ANALYSIS (PER SERVING)
512 Calories (kcal), 29 g Protein, 27 g Carbohydrates, 30 g Fat, 6 g Saturated Fat, 1 g Total Dietary Fibre

Spinach Salad

You can purchase precooked chicken breasts in most supermarkets, or cook them yourself as directed here.

2 145 g/5-oz precooked chicken breasts, sliced or diced

1 285-g/10-oz bag fresh spinach leaves

285 g/10 oz thinly sliced strawberries

30 g/1 oz slivered almonds

180 ml/6 fl oz low-fat raspberry vinaigrette

To cook the chicken: Preheat the oven to 200°C (400°F, gas 6). Line a baking sheet or pie pan with aluminum foil coated with cooking spray. Place the chicken breast(s) on the foil. Season as desired – garlic powder, dried oregano, salt and ground black pepper are good. Bake 10 to 15 minutes or until the chicken is no longer pink inside. Allow to cool before you slice or dice for the salad.

To assemble the salad: Place everything except the chicken in a large bowl and toss to coat with the vinaigrette. Split the salad onto two plates. Arrange the chicken slices or chunks on top of the salads.

Makes 2 servings.

RECIPE NUTRIENT ANALYSIS (PER SERVING)
514 Calories (kcal), 47 g Protein, 13 g Carbohydrates, 30 g Fat, 5 g Saturated Fat, 6 g Total Dietary Fibre

'I looked great for my wedding.'

NAME: MATTHEW KEENER

AGE: 30

OCCUPATION: MEDICAL STUDENT

Medical school had taken its toll on Matthew Keener. A competitive rower, cyclist and runner during his undergraduate years, he found it difficult to organize an exercise regime around a gruelling medical school schedule.

The long hours kept him from eating healthily or regularly. He experienced wild fluctuations in energy levels. At one point, during a surgical rotation, he almost fell asleep at the operating table while watching a procedure.

When he began the Core programme, he discovered that the nutrition philosophies meshed with what he was learning at medical school.

'I knew from studying the glycaemic index that having three large meals and nothing in between would wreak havoc on me,' he said. 'Not only that, but it causes you to pack on the weight instead of building muscle or maintaining your existing lean muscle mass.'

Once a rock-solid, 1.95-metre (6-foot-5), 86-kilogram (190-pound) triathlete, Keener had become a soft 190-pounder, literally a starving student. With his fiancée handling the bulk of their wedding preparations, he decided it was time to do some planning of his own to meet the demands of his busy schedule.

Keener set out time each week to assemble ready-to-go meals. He made sure he had plenty of meal-replacement drinks and bars on hand at all times in case he wanted a snack. 'The bars have been lifesavers,' he says. 'I can throw them in my white coat or backpack and no matter how busy I get, I can always quickly eat one of those.'

The programme forced him to plot out his week in advance. 'If I knew I wasn't going to be near a gym for 2 days, I knew I could still use the physioball I have at home and do some Movement Prep.' (To learn more, see part 3.) 'It was just a matter of spending half an hour to set the schedule for the week.'

The Core Workout, along with better nutrition, gave Keener consistent energy and mental focus throughout the day. Core training also solved a nagging rotator cuff injurythat he had suffered during a skiing accident years before.

By the day of his wedding, 21 August, 2004, Keener was a lean 93 kilograms (205 pounds). 'I looked great for my wedding,' says Keener, who graduated in 2005 and plans to pursue a career in psychiatry. 'But more importantly, I've been able to keep that lean weight on and now have a programme in place that will keep me on track no matter how busy I become in the future as a doctor.'

Prawn and Asparagus

8 asparagus spears

2 lemons

285 g/10 oz defrosted precooked prawns (see note)

1 tsp low-sodium seafood seasoning

1 tbsp extra virgin olive oil

Salt and ground black pepper to taste

Remove the tough bottoms of the asparagus stalks by holding them in both hands and bending until they break. Discard the tough portions and chop each tender portion into three pieces. Set aside. Juice each lemon into separate containers and set these aside. Sprinkle the prawns with the seafood seasoning and set aside. Heat a large sauté pan to medium-high. Add the olive oil and the reserved asparagus. Toss for about 2 minutes. Add the juice of 1 lemon, and toss in the pan for 1 more minute. Create a circle in the middle of the pan and add the prawns. Toss the prawns and asparagus together briefly, then cover and steam for 1 to 2 minutes, until all of the prawns are heated through. Season with salt and pepper to taste. Add the remaining lemon juice, if desired.

Note: *To defrost prawns safely, place them in the fridge overnight.*

Makes 1 serving.

RECIPE NUTRIENT ANALYSIS (PER SERVING)
420 Calories (kcal), 62 g Protein, 25 g Carbohydrates, 17 g Fat, 3 g Saturated Fat, 3 g Total Dietary Fibre

Taco Salad or Soft Tacos

In this recipe, you cook enough meat for 4 servings. You can serve them all at once, or refrigerate 3 servings' worth of cooked meat and leftover vegetables for later.

1 tbsp extra virgin olive oil

570 g/1¼ lb lean minced turkey

1 packet prepackaged taco seasoning

1 large tomato, diced

120 g/4 oz low-fat grated Cheddar cheese (four 30-g/1-oz servings)

1 large avocado, diced at serving time

120 g/4 oz sour cream

120 g/4 oz natural yogurt (four 60-g/2-oz servings)

240 g/8 oz salsa (four 60-g/2-oz servings)

If making the salad:

4 heads romaine lettuce (1 head per serving)

1 425-g/15-oz tin black beans, drained and rinsed

1 285-g/10-oz package defrosted frozen broccoli florets

If making the tacos:

4 25-cm/10-in tortillas (1 per serving). Choose high-fibre tortillas if available

1 head romaine lettuce (about 8 leaves, shredded; optional)

To cook the turkey: Put the oil in a large sauté pan, heat over medium-high heat and add the turkey, following the directions on the taco seasoning packet to cook and season the meat. When the turkey is no longer pink, remove it from the heat and set aside. If saving it for later, then refrigerate immediately.

To make 1 serving of salad: Chop 1 head of the lettuce and place it in a large salad bowl. Top with ¼ of the tinned black beans, ¼ of the tomato, ¼ of the broccoli florets and 30 g/1 oz of the cheese. (To make 4 salads, quadruple these amounts.) Refrigerate until ready to serve. At serving time, add ¼ of the avocado to each salad, then spoon ¼ of the turkey meat over the top of each. Garnish each with 120 g/4 oz of the sour cream mixed with yogurt and 60 g/2 oz of salsa.

To make 1 taco: Microwave 1 soft tortilla on high power for 30 seconds or until soft enough to roll. Place the tortilla on a flat surface and spoon ¼ of the turkey meat down the centre of the tortilla. Top with ¼ of the tomato, 2 shredded lettuce leaves (if desired), 30 g/1 oz of grated cheese and ¼ of the diced avocado. (To make 4 tacos, quadruple these amounts.) Roll up each tortilla and serve each with 60 g/2 oz of sour cream and yogurt mix and 60 g/2 oz of salsa.

Makes 4 taco salads or 4 soft tacos.

TACO SALAD RECIPE NUTRIENT ANALYSIS (PER SERVING)
566 Calories (kcal), 54 g Protein, 21 g Carbohydrates, 30 g Fat, 13 g Saturated Fat, 8 g Total Dietary Fibre
SOFT TACO RECIPE NUTRIENT ANALYSIS (PER SERVING)
716 Calories (kcal), 63g Protein, 61g Carbohydrates, 24g Fat, 6g Saturated Fat, 13g Total Dietary Fibre

CORE SNACKS:
EAT BETWEEN PERIODS

If you've ever attended a sporting event, you've probably snacked throughout the game. After all, 3 hours is a long time to go without eating. Not wanting to miss any of the action, you wait until half-time to find a snack.

Though there are few healthy options available at the stadium, at least you're staying fuelled. Ironically, people tend to nourish themselves more for spectator sports than they do for the Game of Life, where they endure long stretches of the workday with little fuel.

From a young age, many of us were taught to avoid eating between meals. We'll get fat and, at the very least, spoil our dinners. That's what a generation of mums led us to believe.

Actually, spoiling dinner is not such a bad thing if it means you won't overeat, as most people do. You need to keep your blood sugar levels consistent to minimize overeating. The only way to do this is to eat a small meal every 2½ to 3 hours.

Of course, we don't want to consume the equivalent of stadium food. As with your meals, you want your snacks to include a combination of high-fibre carbohydrates, proteins and fats. You could have a cup of cottage cheese or low-fat yogurt (with no added sugar). You could have a piece of fruit with peanut butter, and a handful of nuts. A little tuna or chicken combined with a fruit or vegetable is a good snack.

For some people, there might be little

difference between their meals and their snacks. Breakfasts, lunches and dinners might be smaller than what you've traditionally eaten, since you are no longer trying to eat enough to curb your appetite for the next 6 to 12 hours.

Then again, the size of your meals might remain consistent, with your snacks being somewhat modest. That's okay, too, as long as snacks contain protein, high-fibre carbs and good fats. For time and convenience, you might want to have a protein shake or a high-protein meal-replacement bar.

The challenge with meal-replacement bars is to find something that tastes good and is good for you. Look at the label carefully. Your goal is to find something with 15 to 30 grams of protein, 8 to 20 grams of carbs and a few grams of fat.

You have snacks or shakes built into your schedule three times a day. You might find the late-afternoon feeding the most important, since people tend to feel most sluggish at that time.

For your final snack at night, find something that will stay with you, since it will be a long time before you eat again. Some chicken or fish left over from dinner would be a good snack; a protein shake would also work, as would an apple with peanut butter. Whatever you choose, look for something with plenty of fibre.

So don't feel guilty about those between-meal snacks. In fact, look at them not as guilty pleasures but as essential components of a healthy lifestyle.

CORE SUPPLEMENTS

Walk into any health food shop and you'll find a dizzying array of products that promise to transform your body. For simplicity, we're not going to bother with most of them in this book.

You already know that I recommend a pre-workout shooter or post-workout recovery mix, and shakes as snacks. It's also a good idea to take a multivitamin in the morning, along with an antioxidant complex, which is chock-full of vitamins and minerals.

If you're eating well and following this programme, you can get by without antioxidant supplementation. But even elite athletes who come to Athletes' Performance and have their blood analysed almost always are deficient in some antioxidants. We immediately put them on supplements, and here's why: whenever our bodies endure stress – whether from physical activity, sun damage, pollution or the day-to-day demands of families and jobs – we suffer cellular damage. It's unavoidable. Those damaged cells are known as free radicals. We want to minimize their impact and get them out of our systems immediately.

Think of free radicals as rugby players fighting. Antioxidants are the referees that escort them to the penalty box. They maintain order amongst your cells and slow the ageing process. You can find bottles of antioxidants at a health food shop or supermarket. We recommend a product called Vitrin to our athletes. Though it's more expensive than some antioxidants and only available online, two Vitrin

THE DESK DRAWER PLAYER

One of the biggest obstacles to eating right and maintaining optimal energy is dealing with the hunger pangs that hit throughout the day, especially in an office setting.

Well, no matter what our mums said, between-meal snacks, or 'planned grazing', is the only way to properly fuel your body. This doesn't mean stuffing your face all day long, but instead it means planning what you snack on at specific points throughout the day. .

The last thing you want to do is resort to a vending machine, which is why I keep a desk drawer stocked with healthy food options. I have a box of oatmeal, tear-open packaged tuna fish, apples, oranges and *healthy* snack bars. There's a jar of almonds, a loaf of wholemeal bread, condiments in one-serving packs, a jar of sugar-free applesauce, plastic utensils, paper plates and hand wipes. I have one of those mini-fridges near my desk and I keep it full of bottled water, fresh veggie snacks, fat-free yogurt with no sugar added and ready-to-drink products.

Your 'drawer' doesn't literally have to be in the office. It could be a container you keep in the car, or part of a nappy bag if you're a busy parent. This space has become the key player of my nutrition programme since it often saves me from making bad nutritional choices or trying to get through an afternoon hungry.

No matter how busy I am – and like many people, I find there are times when I can't leave my desk because of constant phone calls, meetings and e-mails – I know that I'll be okay because of the trusty drawer, which I restock periodically. It's not just for snacks; there are adequate supplies for breakfast or lunch if I need it.

Encourage your colleagues, employees and boss to create their own drawers. It will raise office productivity by keeping energy high and eliminating lengthy mid-afternoon breaks to hunt for snacks. You'll set an example, thus elevating others. Most important, it will keep everyone on track with a healthy nutritional programme.

---

caplets contain 29 essential vitamins and minerals, plus the antioxidant equivalent of five servings of fruits and vegetables.

There's been a lot of concern in recent years about supplements, much of it well-deserved. There's stuff you can buy legally in a health food shop that I strongly caution our athletes against taking, either because of anecdotal evidence that suggests it's harmful or because no long-term studies have been conducted on the effects. With this in mind, I recommend that you stick to the supplemental foods recommended in this book.

Chapter 6 Summary: To eat healthily and consistently, start thinking of meal preparation as quick 'meal assembly' involving a lean protein source, colour- and fibre-rich carbohydrates and healthy fats.

CORE MEAL ASSEMBLY

By now, your shopping trolley should be bulging with foods that taste great and are full of nutrients. The biggest misperception about eating right is that your meals have to be bland and boring. Nothing could be further from the truth. By using just the items mentioned below – and in earlier chapters – you can produce dozens of rich, tasty meals.

I'm not suggesting that you give up your favourite recipes. Many people are talented in the kitchen, and one of the joys of life is sharing a leisurely meal with friends and family. But there's often not enough time to prepare an elaborate meal.

The key is to stop looking at cooking in terms of complicated and lengthy preparation and instead view it as meal 'assembly'. Take a lean protein source, like turkey or lean beef, some carbohydrates rich in colour and fibre, and some nutritious fats and you've got a great meal.

SERVING SIZE GUIDE

This list can serve as a basic guide when you're substituting one form of food for another. Remember that whole foods are always better for you than processed foods.

Vegetables: 185 g/6½ oz raw veggies, 90 g/3 oz cooked veggies, 150 ml/¼ pint vegetable juice, 170 g/6 oz cooked dry beans

Fruits: 1 medium-size fruit (1 medium apple or medium pear), 150 g/5½ oz canned or chopped fruit, or 150 ml/¼ pint fruit juice

Breads and Cereals: 1 slice of bread, 40 g/1¼ oz ready-to-eat cereal, 170 g/6 oz cooked rice or pasta

Protein: 115 g/4 oz meat (the size of a pack of cards), a handful of nuts, 2 tbsp peanut butter

Fats: 1 tbsp olive oil, rapeseed (canola) oil or flaxseed (linseed) oil

Dairy Products: 240 ml/8 fl oz milk, 150 g/5½ oz cottage cheese, 30 g/1 oz or 1 slice of cheese

BREAKFAST

Carbohydrates
● Choose two items.
60 g/2 oz Kashi cereal or wholegrain cereal
1 piece of wholemeal bread (no enriched flour)
1 grapefruit
45 g/1½ oz porridge oats
75 g/2½ oz grapes
75 g/2½ oz cantaloupe
40 g/3 oz honeydew melon
200 g/7 oz low-fat, low-sugar yogurt
45 g/1½ oz wholegrain bran cereal

Protein
● Choose one or two items.
4 egg whites
egg substitute equivalent to 2 eggs
2 eggs
150 g/5½ oz cottage cheese
240 ml/8 fl oz skimmed milk
3 slices deli meat
2 tablespoons peanut butter

Vegetables
● Choose as many as you like.
90 g/3 oz broccoli
30 g/1 oz spinach
100 g/3½ oz green beans
170 g/6 oz tomatoes
125 g/4½ oz cucumbers
45 g/1½ oz romaine lettuce
100 g/3½ oz mushrooms
200 g/7 oz tomato sauce

Healthy Fats
● Choose one item.
1 tbsp flaxseed (linseed) oil
1 to 2 tbsp olive oil
1 to 2 tbsp rapeseed (canola) oil
45 g/1½ oz low-fat cheese
30 g/1 oz dry-roasted nuts

Sample Breakfast
60 g/2 oz Kashi cereal and an omelette made with 4 egg whites, veggies, and 45 g/1½ oz low-fat cheese.

- Plan, plan, plan.
- Control the clock.
- Protein + Carbs + Healthy fats.
- Eat to live. Don't live to eat.

Lunch and dinner need not be major productions, especially since you're eating more often. Just take some fish, chicken or lean red meat; add some vegetables, fruit, or both; and wash it down with two glasses of cold water, or even a glass of red wine. There you have it: a good meal.

As we mentioned earlier, you can cook plenty of chicken and fish on Saturdays or Sundays. Buy some prepackaged salads. Put together some vegetables and fruits. The key is to have things ready so you won't be left scrambling for food, which inevitably results in poor nutritional choices.

The following is a handy guide to assembling your meals and eating properly. It's not an exhaustive list – we provided even more options earlier in this section – but it does give you everything you need to assemble nutritious meals in the least amount of time.

LUNCH OR DINNER

Protein
● Choose one or two items.
115 g/4 oz grilled chicken
150 g/5½ oz cottage cheese
1 can tuna packed in water
115 g/4 oz skinless turkey
115 g/4 oz lean pork (grilled)
115 g/4 oz grilled lean red meat

Carbohydrates
● Choose one or two.
170 g/6 oz brown rice
200 g/7 oz whole wheat pasta
170 g/6 oz long grain wild rice
1 wholemeal roll
1 slice wholemeal bread

Vegetables
● Choose as many as you like.
90 g/3 oz broccoli
30 g/1 oz spinach
100 g/3½ oz green beans
170 g/6 oz tomatoes
125 g/4½ oz cucumbers
45 g/1½ oz romaine lettuce
100 g/3½ oz mushrooms
200 g/7 oz tomato sauce

Beans and Pulses
● Choose one.
170 g/6 oz black beans
170 g/6 oz haricot beans
170 g/6 oz pinto beans
170 g/6 oz kidney beans

Low-Glycaemic Fruits
● Choose one or two.
1 apple
1 peach
1 plum
75 g/2½ oz cherries
1 grapefruit
1 pear

Healthy Fats
● Choose one item.
1 to 2 tbsp olive oil
1 to 2 tbsp rapeseed (canola) oil
45 g/1½ oz cheese
30 g/1 oz dry-roasted nuts
(e.g. almonds)

Sample Lunch or Dinner
170 g/6 oz brown rice and 170 g/ 6 oz grilled chicken, with a side salad made from 60 g/2 oz spinach and 125 g/4½ oz cucumber with 2 tbsp *each* olive oil and vinegar.

CHAPTER 7

ROAD GAMES

t's always more difficult for a sports team to win on the road than it is at home. After all, the athletes must face the grind of travel, playing in a hostile environment and not having all of the creature comforts of home.

To compensate, teams stay at the nicest hotels, bring planeloads of equipment and implement a game plan tailored specifically to the task. The idea is to control the unfamiliar environment as much as possible. Still, in order to succeed and win the game, the team must play at a higher level at an opponent's venue. There's little margin for error.

The same is true with nutrition. It's less of a challenge to eat right at home. After all, you've created a home ground advantage by stocking your fridge and cupboards with healthy foods and ensuring you keep healthy food at work. You've plotted your meals and snacks around work and weekly routines. You've put your family on notice that you're going to eat healthily – hopefully getting them to buy into the same programme.

Away from home, however, it's much more difficult to eat right. Whether it's a busy day of commitments and errands running around town, a business trip involving air travel and hotel stays, or simply visiting a friend's house for an evening, you will face formidable obstacles to eating right.

So, once again, you should be proactive and plan ahead. At the very least, grab bottled water, fruit and a bag of nuts before leaving the house. Keep healthy meal-replacement bars in the car, or in your briefcase or bag. If you're going to be running around all day, pack a healthy salad or a one-serving plastic container with a lean protein source and a vegetable.

In order to stay properly fuelled, you must eat roughly every 3 hours, and that's a challenge away from home. We've already discussed how to handle eating at work – think of that key player drawer and bringing lunch from home – but that's a little easier since work routines are fairly consistent.

There's nothing more counterproductive to a healthy lifestyle than playing goalie when it comes to nutrition. If you're out running errands, chances are you're in a hurry. You lose track of time and the next thing you know, you're popping into a corner shop or snack bar in search of quick nourishment.

Not only does this wreak havoc on your body but it's also time-consuming, expensive and frustrating. You don't want to have to pay for the right to eat bad food, and waste time doing it. Plan ahead and you'll save yourself both time and money while fuelling your body for maximum energy.

Travelling presents another challenge. In recent years, some airlines have eliminated meal service, which is a good thing because it keeps us from eating highly processed airline food and forces us to be proactive about meal planning. Instead of buying expensive pizza and junk food in the concourse or eating airline food, bring a meal from home. Don't forget the bottled water.

On long car trips, fill a cooler with bottled water, fresh fruit, vegetables, lean protein sources, healthy snack bars and low-fat, low-sugar yogurt. Snack in the car and stop at rest areas instead of pulling off the motorway and frequenting fast-food joints. Again, you'll save time and money in addition to making sure you are eating right.

For longer trips, whether by car or plane, be sure to take meal-replacement powder to mix into a shake. If you're travelling, instead of lugging around a blender, a far better choice is to use a specifically designed shaker bottle, which gives you a rotator cuff workout in the process! (They're available at many health food shops and also online.) Fill a small plastic container with your whey protein, which you can sprinkle onto porridge to punch up the protein content, and mix with water and juice for pre-workout shooters. Be sure to pack multivitamins and antioxidants too.

Eating in sit-down restaurants need not be challenging. It's almost always possible to order grilled chicken or fish with vegetables and a salad. Skip the bread and creamy appetizers.

If a menu item isn't quite right, you usually have the option of substituting or asking for it to be prepared differently.

No matter what kind of 'road game' you encounter, control the environment as much as possible. Plan ahead. Bring all of the equipment you need; it need not weigh you down. Let those other travellers stand in line at the airport for a greasy piece of pizza. Let others waste their time, money and possibly even their health at the road-side fast food restaurants.

We'll talk in the coming chapters about strategies to work out on the road, which people generally find easier than eating right when travelling. But whether it's exercise or nutrition, you can take pride in knowing that you've brought the home ground advantage with you.

THE TOUGHEST ROAD GAME

There are certain sporting venues that make it almost impossible for a visiting team to win. Whether it's a freezing cold playing field or a

BEING A GRACIOUS GUEST

When it comes to nutrition, it's tough to be a gracious guest. Sooner or later, you'll find yourself at a family gathering facing a heaped plate of Aunt Edna's lasagne, buttery garlic bread and mashed potatoes. Or maybe the boss or a key client has invited you over for spaghetti, roast pork or some other fat-laden dish.

I suppose you could fake an upset stomach or declare your allegiance to a special diet, which would be partially true. But either way, you're probably going to offend someone.

Your best bet is to eat a small portion, which will be easier if you're eating six meals a day. Not only that, but you should eat before arriving at the House of Fat. That way you'll feel full and not be inclined to down a bad meal just because it's put in front of you.

It's easier to get by at a casual party. Nobody is going to notice if you don't touch the crisps, dips, pizza, burgers, hot dogs, beer and fizzy drinks. Like the sit-down dinner situation, it's best to plan ahead and eat before the party or bring dishes to share.

Of course, you could schedule your free day to coincide with the party, which might be the easiest solution. But sometimes there are too many events and not enough free days.

Planning ahead is the best strategy. After all, when it comes to nutrition, sometimes a friendly environment can be hostile territory.

home crowd that taunts opposing teams, it's tough to win on the road.

The same is true with nutrition. On the road, it's more difficult to eat right. You're generally at the mercy of restaurant menus, and you're usually pressed for time. Ideally, you can still find a healthier restaurant, but there will be times when you end up in the fast-food joint.

When you enter the opposing venue and see its vast menu of unhealthy yet tempting foods, don't forget your goals: *peak performance and optimal health.* Fast-food restaurants can be a roadblock to your nutrition goals, but with a little planning and some specific requests, you can turn any fast-food-restaurant meal into one that is healthier. Just remember these specific rules, courtesy of our wonderful Amanda Carlson, the nutrition manager and research co-ordinator at Athletes' Performance:

1. Stay away from the fryer (e.g., fried chicken, chips, etc). Choose a side salad or baked potato as your side.

2. Go with grilled foods instead.

3. The less legs the better. Grilled chicken or fish is a healthier option than a burger.

4. Remove the skin. If there is skin on your chicken or turkey, take it off.

5. Hold the mayo.

6. Go with water instead of fizzy drinks. Not only is it better for you, it's free.

Think about what you have already eaten throughout the day. Make choices that are low in fat and that contain the right amount of carbohydrates for you. Remember that carbohydrates equal fuel, so if it is earlier in the day or after a workout, you may need more of them. If it is later in the day and less activity is planned, then a reduced amount will do just fine. Consider the following tips to help reduce the amount of processed carbohydrates in your meal:

1. Remove the bun from your burger or chicken sandwich, or remove just the top and eat it open-faced.

2. Order an extra chicken breast for your salad and skip the bun.

3. Leave the croutons off your salad.

Now, let's take a look at some of the world's toughest venues in which to eat properly and how to make the choices. This list notes the best options offered.

Fast-food outlets

● Salad with a low-fat dressing

● Grilled chicken sandwich and a side salad with a low-fat dressing

● Large chilli with a side salad with low-fat dressing

● Small chilli and a baked potato with steamed broccoli

- If you must eat a cheeseburger, choose a single with cheese – and don't add any mayo or other creamy sauce

- Include water with these items. If you must have a fizzy drink, always try to choose diet

Mexican

  Choose grilled fish or meat dishes, with salsa and salads

  Avoid sour cream, nachos, tacos and cheese

- Choose healthy fillings for tortillas

Indian

- Choose a wholewheat roti or chapati rather than naan, which is made with white flour and is full of fat

  If possible, order a serving of steamed vegetables to accompany the meal

  Avoid korma and masala dishes, as these are made with cream

  Choose plain boiled rice rather than pilau rice, which is cooked with fat

  As a rule, choose drier dishes rather than those with a lot of sauce

  Tikka dishes can be a good choice, as can those dishes based on vegetables rather than meat

Chinese

- Choose plain steamed rice rather than egg fried rice

- Avoid battered dishes

- Avoid deep fried dishes such as spring rolls

- Choose some vegetable dishes, such as steamed pak choi (bok choy)

- Choose fish rather than red meat where possible

Italian

- Don't order garlic bread

- Choose pasta sauces that are not cream based, classic tomato-based sauces such as Napolitana are a good choice

- Avoid cheesy lasagne and similar dishes

- If you drink wine with your meal, be sure to also drink water

Sandwich bars

- Choose any healthy options advertised

- Choose low-fat dressings

- There's no reason to go light on mustard, but avoid butter and creamy dressings like mayonaise and salad cream

- Avoid cheese and the fattier sliced meats – lean turkey can be a good choice

Cafés

● Ask for skimmed milk in your coffee

● Avoid adding sugar to your tea or coffee

● If you want a snack, choose a small salad rather than a slice of cake

● Drink a glass of water with your coffee

Subway

● Choose a six-inch turkey, roast beef, chicken or ham sub on wholemeal bread, or go for a wrap

● Make your sandwich into a salad

● Skip the cheese

● Add plenty of vegetables such as tomatoes, pickles, black olives, cucumbers and green peppers

● Go light on the mayonnaise

● Drink water instead of fizzy drinks

Pizzerias

● Choose a thin-crust vegetable, Hawaiian or seafood pizza

● Add grilled chicken, ham and veggies

● Do not order garlic bread

● Order a salad with low-fat dressing on the side instead

● Ask for less cheese

● Order water with your meal

McDonald's

● Chicken Salad Toasted Deli Sandwich on brown bread

● Chicken Tikka Toasted Deli Sandwich on brown bread

● Grilled chicken Caesar salad with ½ packet low-fat balsamic vinaigrette instead of Caesar dressing

● Cheeseburger (if you must) with a side salad topped with ½ packet of low-fat balsamic vinaigrette

● Egg McMuffin

Sit-Down Restaurants

● Choose grilled chicken or fish

● If choosing a steak, trim the fat and choose cuts with less marbling

● Start with a salad with low-fat dressing

● Choose steamed vegetables as sides

● Eat rolls and potato dishes in moderation

● Try to avoid dishes with creamy sauces

● Ask for sauces and dressings on the side so you can control the amount you use

An overall lifestyle of healthy choices improves health and performance. Long-term healthy eating habits overpower one not-so-great choice. The occasional lapse in your diet will not undo the progress you have made by following the Core Nutrition programme.

Chapter 7 Summary: Eating on the road presents a number of challenges. The key, once again, is proper planning. Stock your car, desk, briefcase, handbag or nappy bag with healthy options so you won't have to turn to junk food when things get hectic. You need not eat poorly at sit-down restaurants. There are usually some healthy options on the menu. Go with grilled chicken or fish and steamed vegetables. If you must eat at a fast-food restaurant, make the best possible choice that you can.

CORE
MOVEMENT

BUILDING YOUR INNER CORE

When you people-watch at the shopping centre or airport, it's easy to tell who's in shape and who's not. We make the same judgements when we look at ourselves in the mirror. If you are committed to the Core programme, your body will undergo a physical transformation. But I need you to think not just in terms of the way you look but also in terms of the way you *move*.

When I watch people, the first thing I notice is their movement patterns. I might see them walking with one or both of their feet rotating outwards, which prevents them from rolling over on their toes or using their ankle joints. That leads to tight ankles, hips and lower-back pain.

Other times, I notice a person's hip instability. With every step they take, they put undue stress upon and cause excess wear of the knees, feet, groin and, by extension, the spine.

In the short term, this might not seem like anything other than soreness after a long day of walking. Down the road, however, one of those areas will become a major problem.

These people, some of whom are in decent shape, suffer from 'biomechanical dysfunction'. From a height/weight standpoint, they might look like they're in above-average condition, but they still have biomechanical dysfunction because they no longer can perform the necessary movements to thrive and sustain a high quality of life. Maybe they don't realize it now, but they will when something breaks down. It's like driving your car when the wheels aren't aligned.

At our training centres we conduct an analysis of each athlete's movement-pattern efficiency. The idea is to make sure they meet and exceed the excruciating demands of their sports. We also take a look at the athletes' software – in other words, *their brains*. The Game of Life installs viruses into our software through injury and illness, lack of activity and improper training. We need to improve the way our software boots up so that our bodies operate efficiently to create functional, fluid movement that protects and propels us.

We do this by trying to determine which, if any, muscles are 'overfiring', creating tightness and tension, and by seeing whether any muscles have been turned off all together. This causes other muscles to overcompensate, leading to muscle fatigue and strain.

When we get these movement patterns working properly, we find a body that is perfectly balanced to efficiently store and release energy with every step. These graceful patterns allow muscles to complement one another, smoothly transferring energy back and forth; they feed off one another in perfect harmony. This programme will help you to achieve the same feeling.

Most exercise programmes provide the type of workout that you equate with traditional fitness. Many people see exercise solely in the one-dimensional, old-school mode. Authors and followers of such programmes might belittle you for your willingness to try something new, going beyond the stale, inefficient regimes at the gym. But by using the Core programme, you will be able to more efficiently reach your fitness goals than the majority of people exercising at clubs – and often more efficiently than their trainers, who believe people should follow the same programme they use every day.

The movements you'll learn through the Core programme might seem unusual, but they're effective. They are derivatives of the guiding principles we use at Athletes' Performance. We can't take credit for these powerful movements because they are merely variations of childhood movement; they just need dusting off.

As a baby, you started to learn these movement patterns, first by rolling over. Gradually, you began to crawl, stand, squat, walk and run. You progressed during the preteen and teenage years, refining these movement patterns to higher levels. And then what happened? You stopped progressing, falling into a less active lifestyle of school, work and screen time. That is where you left off, and that's where we will begin.

At first, this programme might seem remedial as we return to the basics of movement, but be patient. Don't get frustrated as you learn these new exercises. Give yourself time.

Have you written down a consistent, weekly plan that is realistic given your time constraints?

Do you define the success of your exercise programme primarily by the changes you see in the mirror?

Do you know how your programme improves your body function so that you can thrive given the demands of the Game of Life?

Does your programme create pain as much as, if not more than, it reduces pain?

Does travel, the demands of your job or family, or another external factor throw you off of your programme?

Like a baby, we will learn and steadily progress throughout your lifespan.

We have broken up these exercises into four simple categories:

- Movement Preparation (or 'Movement Prep')
- Prehabilitation (or 'Prehab')
- Strength and Performance Circuits
- Cardio

These four categories or 'players' are important individually and even more so as a comprehensive regime. They might have you off-balance at first, but the athlete inside you will adjust to meet the challenge.

In part 4, we will add a fifth element called Regeneration. Think of Regeneration as a substitute in rugby or football – the player who comes in fresh and scores the deciding try or goal. This element will allow you to catch your breath, and it will encourage all the benefits of the four preceding elements to take effect. That way, when I call you back into the game,

you will be able to improve on your last performance and make even more progress.

First, I want you to toss aside everything you know about exercise. The problem with most workout routines is that they're based on bodybuilding. You work your biceps and triceps on one day, your legs the next. But unless your goals are to take up residence in a gym and win bodybuilding championships, you're wasting time and not improving overall health. Before you get started, take the time to answer questions in the Core Movement Assessment above.

In this chapter, you will learn to adopt a realistic exercise plan that you'll be able to stick to regardless of the demands of work, family and travel. You'll see why it does not make sense to define fitness by how you look in the mirror but rather by your body's function and how resistant it is to injury and long-term deterioration.

Like the rest of the programme, we want to focus on the centred self and build from the inside out. Not only that, but we're now thinking of ourselves as athletes, and athletes do not train with the intent of improving their looks. They train in order to master the movements that their sport requires. We need to train the same way to compete in the Game of Life.

You might think that your daily movements do not require much athleticism – but oh, how wrong you are. What about lifting children or shopping? What about reacting quickly and maintaining balance when you slip on a wet floor? How about climbing stairs, rushing to grab a taxi or bus, or working in the garden?

All of these things require athletic, *functional* movement. If you're going to invest the time to work out, why not do it with more than aesthetics in mind? By following the Core Workout and Nutrition programme, you'll train your body, and as an added bonus, you'll get in phenomenal shape – in far less time than bodybuilders spend in the gym.

Bodybuilding-based workouts view the physique as a series of parts, and most people tend to think of movement as starting from the limbs. If we reach out to grab something or step forwards, we think of those motions as originating with the end result – we've reached out, therefore, we've used our arms.

But movement starts from the very centre of the body, the core area of the torso. That's why we refer to the torso as the *pillar* – it's the structural centre of movement and life. The way we maintain that pillar – its alignment and function – directly correlates to the health of our organs and the rest of our bodies. Everything is interrelated.

PILLAR STRENGTH

Pillar strength is the foundation of all movement. It consists of hip, core and shoulder stability. (If you're having a hard time getting your head around this concept, it might help to picture your body as a mannequin with no limbs.) Those three areas give us a centre axis from which to move. If you think of the body as a wheel, the pillar is the hub and the limbs are spokes.

We want to have the hub perfectly aligned so we can draw energy from it and effectively transfer that energy throughout the body. It's impossible to move the limbs efficiently and forcefully if they're not attached to something solid and stable.

There's a reason why parents are forever telling kids to sit up straight. Without pillar strength, without what I call 'perfect posture', you will significantly increase the potential for injury in a chain that starts with your lower back, descends all the way to the knees and ankles, and rises up to your neck, shoulders and elbows.

The reason we train body *movements* instead of parts is because everything about the body's engineering is connected. What happens to the big toe affects the knees, the hips and ultimately the shoulders. The muscular system is both complex and simple, a series of muscular and fascial bands that work seamlessly to produce efficient movement. Many workout programmes do more damage than good by producing muscle imbalances and inefficient movement patterns that sabotage this highly co-ordinated operating system that we're born with.

Remember the way that movement evolves in infants. They move on their backs until one day this action allows them to roll over, initiating the hip crossover movement. Soon they progress to crawling, standing and, finally, walking. With each step, they realize how to stabilize their bodies.

Ageing reverses that process. Many people lose the ability to squat and maintain their balance, creating poor posture. Eventually, they lose the ability to stand, surrendering the core fundamental movement patterns they developed as toddlers. But instead of conceding that devolution as an unavoidable part of ageing, why not look at getting older as a process of taking these movements to new levels? In this programme, you're going to take your body to the highest levels of performance and movement capabilities by challenging yourself to increase flexibility and stability. We'll help you do this by adding resistance or increasing the balance demands. This will put you further and further away from the regression of ageing.

Look, I'm not here to bash bodybuilding and tell you not to lift weights. This programme includes resistance training because of its undeniable benefits. The Movement Prep and Prehab routines you'll learn are not a tricksy programme to ram the concept of functional exercise down your throat. It's more about reprogramming the body to function properly – as nature intended – and to continually become stronger. It's possible to become physically stronger every day of our lives.

Instead of looking at movement as coming out of the arms and legs, remember this perfect posture. If you can master the following three elements of pillar strength – shoulder stability, core stability and hip stability – both while working out and in everyday movement, you will go a long way towards a healthier life.

SHOULDER STABILITY

Anyone who participates in a sport involving hitting or throwing understands the importance of the rotator cuff. It's even more important in everyday life.

We tend to think of the hands and arms as carrying the workload for the upper body, but it's really the shoulder, or at least it should be. After all, we think of someone *shouldering* a burden, not 'arming' one.

The shoulder 'girdle' consists of the humerus, scapula and clavicle. It's engineered for a remarkable range of three-dimensional movement. From the shoulder, it's possible to rotate, press and pull. We can raise our arms to the side or across the body. We can rotate shoulders by holding the elbows in and by moving the hands up and in – or in a 90-degree angle to the torso.

Our natural instinct is to drop the shoulders forwards, especially after long periods of sitting.

THE AMISH WORKOUT?

You probably wouldn't think of the Amish, a conservative religious group who live in some parts of the United States and Canada, as a very athletic people. But because they work mostly as farmers and shun technology, spending no time in front of computers and televisions, they actually are among the fittest.

A recent study of physical activity and body composition in an Old Order Amish community by the American College of Sports Medicine (ACSM) suggests that a large decline in work-related physical activity is a major contributing factor to the obesity epidemic.

Ninety-eight Amish adults in a southern Ontario farming community wore pedometers and logged their physical activities for 7 days.

Amish men reported an average of 10 hours of vigorous work per week and took an average of 18,425 steps a day. Amish women, most of whom work as homemakers, still logged an average of 14,196 daily steps. On average, the Amish participated in roughly *six times* the amount of weekly physical activity performed by nearly 2,000 participants in a recent survey in 12 nations.

'The Amish were able to show us just how far we've fallen in the last 150 years or so in terms of the amount of physical activity we typically perform,' says David R. Bassett, professor at the University of Tennessee, who served as lead researcher for the study. 'Their lifestyle indicates that physical activity played a critical role in keeping our ancestors fit and healthy.'

The ACSM study found that only 4 per cent of the Amish surveyed were obese and only 26 per cent were overweight. Compare that with the United States, where 31 per cent of adults are obese and 64.5 per cent are overweight.

Because of their high activity levels, the Amish stay fit despite a high-fat, high-sugar diet of meat, potatoes, gravy, eggs, vegetables, bread, pies and cakes.

If you log 10 laborious hours a week pushing a plough or lifting heavy beams, feel free to enjoy the 'Amish Diet'. But wouldn't it be easier to accomplish the same level of fitness by tweaking your diet and spending a lot less time working out?

But you want to do the opposite, bringing the shoulders back and down, which will give you proper posture.

Remember *The Karate Kid*? Mr Miyagi, the wise martial arts instructor, made his young student Daniel LaRusso paint his fence and wax his cars. For days this went on and Daniel wondered if he was ever going to learn karate. When he confronted Miyagi, the old man asked him to demonstrate the various motions of painting and waxing and then attacked Daniel from all angles. Using the same motions, Daniel easily defended himself and quickly realized that he had not just been painting and waxing but stabilizing and strengthening his shoulder muscles and mastering these vital, functional movements.

If you're involved in martial arts, this programme will help by stabilizing your shoulders – and I won't make you wax cars and paint houses. Even if you have no desire to become the next Bruce Lee, you must strengthen this area to perform everyday activities from cleaning to passing objects to filing to, yes, waxing and painting.

Most of us don't realize how hunched over we are from sitting at computers and travelling in cars and aeroplanes. People tend to think that this affects only the elderly, but that's not the case. The next time you're people-watching at an airport, pay attention to the position of their thumbs. If they're rotated in, pointing towards the body, that means their heads and shoulders have moved forwards.

Unless those people do something, I guarantee that they will soon have rotator cuff and back problems, which will limit their ability to participate in the daily activities of life.

As people age, they tend to flex forwards, as if the chest is caving in. We want to do the opposite, almost as if there's a fishhook inserted under the sternum, pulling us up. This will allow the shoulders to fall into place and help to give perfect posture.

We're not trying to be military cadets, standing bolt straight at attention. Instead, think of this as standing or sitting tall in a comfortable position, always elevating the sternum.

The exercises in this programme will require you to bring the shoulders back and down, but you'll want to make it a daily habit. To make lasting change, we want to lengthen the chest and strengthen the muscles of the upper back. Think of pulling your shoulders towards your back pockets. This posture is the exact opposite of the shoulder shrug, the same motion that you make when you say, 'I don't know'. That's what a sitting lifestyle does to you. If you create a habit of bringing your shoulders down, you'll be amazed at the results. People will find you more confident and think you've lost weight because you're no longer slouched over. They might even think you've grown. There have been instances of adults following this programme and gaining up to 25 centimetres (1 inch) of height from standing tall and bringing their shoulders back, as well as improving hip and core stability.

CORE STABILITY

The middle third of our pillar is the 'core', which consists of the muscles of the abdomen, torso and lower back. It's the vital link between shoulder and hip stability, and it includes such muscle groups as the rectus abdominis, transversus abdominis, internal and external obliques, lats, the erector spinae and the many small stabilizer muscles that lie between the vertebrae of the spine, and which help to hold us upright.

These are the tiny muscles that often get shut off because of a back injury and never become reactivated, causing long-term back problems. These small stabilizer muscles cannot function alone; they must be helped by training the muscles of the core to become strong and stable with the right types of recruitment patterns that will enable them to work in tandem with the shoulders and hips.

Core training is *not* just about the abs – abs are less than a third of the equation. Countless books and magazine articles promise great abs, and though many of them have terrific exercises that we believe in, they're of little use unless done in conjunction with exercises aimed at integrating your shoulders and hips.

Instead of just focusing on the abs, we want to create the framework for all movement. The aim isn't just a well-sculpted midsection; it's a high-performance core.

In order to maximize the benefit of the exercises in this book, it's important to keep your tummy tight, not just while exercising but all day. Think of your tummy flat against the hip bones. Keep your tummy tight, as if pulling your belly button off the belt buckle. This isn't the same as sucking in your gut and holding your breath. Keep the abdominals in, but still breathe.

The abdominal and lower-back muscles work as a team. The key player is the transverse abdominis (TA), which is the first muscle that's recruited each time you move. If you can keep that TA activated and your tummy tight, you'll be well on your way to optimum movement and preventing long-term deterioration.

HIP STABILITY

All of those muscles that attach to your ribs and spine are extremely important for shoulder and core stability. But what good would this be without a strong foundation?

In all the people I evaluate, including the best athletes in the world, the number one focus is hip function and stability – in other words, how they use their pelvis. If people better understood how to use the pelvis and hips, we could eradicate lower-back pain, knee pain, foot ailments and a host of other aches that make us miserable.

We tend to think that if our ankles, knees or feet hurt, there must be something wrong with those areas. But if we again look at the body as a wheel, the pillar, and more specifically, the pelvis, is the hub of that wheel. The pelvis is in charge of controlling the spokes. You might have the greatest spokes (legs and thighs), but if something goes wrong with the hub, the spokes cannot function.

Many injuries are caused by hip tightness and a lack of hip stability. As a result, the body does not recruit the necessary muscles from the pelvic region, and it puts more stress on other areas, which overcompensate and get injured.

We want to go to the source of the problem and prevent injuries from happening. On either

'My pain just seemed to dissipate.'

NAME: JAIME MERRIFIELD

AGE: 45

OCCUPATION: VETERINARIAN

Jaime Merrifield was an avid triathlete until she was diagnosed several years ago with three separate health problems – chronic fatigue syndrome, chronic mononucleosis and fibromyalgia, a musculoskeletal pain and fatigue disorder characterized by pain in the muscles, ligaments and tendons.

She's not sure exactly what brought on the health problems, but she has a few ideas. At the age of 11, she dived off her father's shoulders and hit her head on the bottom of a swimming pool. As a young adult, doctors told her she had the spine of a rugby player, so compressed were her vertebrae. She chalked that up to a bicycle accident at the age of 23 and the stress from long hours spent standing as a teacher.

'I would seem healthy and fit and then I'd crash for a month and sleep,' she says. 'People always thought I was lazy, but it turned out that I have these chronic conditions.'

The ailments were devastating for an active working mum in her mid-forties who has a busy schedule as a vet. She had tried other exercise programmes in the past only to give up when the pain became too much. With the Core programme, she found the pain became more manageable. In fact, some of her chronic pain began to dissipate.

'What I like about the programme is the combination of light weights and stretching,' she says. 'The key is the order in which you do them. I've done variations of a lot of it independently, using a physioball and doing Pilates, but this has proven to be the best mix. It's helped so much both mentally and physically.'

Merrifield found the Movement Prep routine especially beneficial.

'You get that endorphin release after the workout, and my pain just seemed to dissipate. I stopped getting so many migraines.'

As a vet and a pain sufferer, Jaime has studied what causes pain and the links to depression.

It's no surprise to find that anyone suffering from chronic pain might feel depressed, but Jaime believes that research in the coming years will show a neurological link between the two.

'People will tell you they suffered depression after a major injury, and that's no coincidence,' she says. 'It's a vicious cycle. I've found there's something in the way the exercises of the Core programme are arranged that has proven, at least for me, to really inhibit those pain triggers.'

As a triathlete, Jaime always valued an active lifestyle, and she suffered when that was taken away from her. Now, she views training as a necessity to get through her days without pain, not just an enjoyable hobby.

'If I miss a day or two, I feel like I don't want to get out of bed', she says. 'If this programme can have this kind of impact on someone like me, I can only imagine the positive effects it could have on other people.'

side of the pelvis is a hip 'capsule', where the femur attaches to the pelvis. This along with more than 40 muscles in and around the hip capsule creates the 'hip cuff'. This should allow you to rotate your knees in or all the way out, as well as lifting your leg up or back and in every combination. You should be able to lift a leg up and across your body in a lunge.

Most people get into trouble squatting by using their quadriceps rather than the muscles of the hips to initiate movement. As a result, the knees slide forwards, the glutes (your buttocks) don't get involved and there's undue pressure on the knees and back. Our goal is to become more glute-dominant. Watch kids and see how well they squat and stand up. Many of us have lost this movement from sitting too much and being inactive.

Thankfully, we can get it back. Let's practise for a moment. From a standing position, place your feet further than hip width apart. Lean forwards, arms straight ahead. Elevate your chest by feeling tall and pulling your shoulders towards the back pockets and keep your tummy tight. Now, try and sit with the hips; instead of flopping down, as you might if there was a chair underneath, sit firmly by using your hips. Try to create an arch in your lower back, shifting the weight to the middle part of your foot, even a little towards the heel. Feel the glutes and the other muscles of your hip capsule stretch as you lower your body. Squeeze your glutes to stand back up.

Now try to push your pelvis forwards while standing and *then* squat. It doesn't work because you end up driving the knees over the toes. No wonder so many people suffer from knee injuries.

We want to initiate all movement from the hips, while maintaining perfect posture. If you're going up steps, squatting to pick something up or simply standing up, squeeze your glutes until your legs are extended. Walk with your toes pointed forwards, your chest over your knee, and push through your hips until your leg is extended. That might mean you have to skip every other step, but that's okay. This way, the pressure is on your hips – where nature intended – not the knees.

The reason we see so many running-related injuries is because people don't have the necessary hip stability. Runners have to be able to effectively balance on a single leg and move from the hips. If the hips don't stabilize, the force created by the pounding of running is stored in the body. That energy is absorbed and stored in the muscles, tendons and joints, leading to overuse injuries.

But if you're stable in the hips, core and shoulders, the energy transfers through the feet, legs, core and through the opposite arm, leading to maximum performance. So, by creating a mobile and stabile hip joint, you will store and release energy efficiently, creating optimum movement.

A properly functioning pair of hip capsules

is the most powerful thing you have in your body, but it's the most destructive if it's locked down. If your hip capsule is locked down, lacking stability and mobility, it's as if a bone is welded to the pelvis – it's like having a cast on your hip. To get anything to move, you need to have excessive motion in your back and knees. But the better job you do of creating stability, mobility and strength around the hip, the less potential there is for injury and the far better chance you'll have of performing well in any activity you undertake.

But the benefit of initiating movement with your hips doesn't stop there. You know the easiest way to get 'buns' of steel? Use them constantly. Don't do just one isolated workout. People who have flat, shapeless buttocks do not use their hips and glutes properly in everyday movement; they just have a couple of saggy bags back there. Look for every opportunity to lengthen and strengthen those glutes, whether it's squatting, going up stairs, getting out of a chair or simply walking. This is the foundation for all movement.

Think of life as one big glute workout and you'll see amazing results. Every time you walk, move and bend, fire (squeeze) those glutes. Don't take them for granted.

One way to keep track of how active you're becoming in your day-to-day life is simply to use a pedometer. These cheap, easy-to-use devices keep track of how many steps you take. At the end of the day, you can see how much you moved – or did not move – and that's terrific motivation to turn your daily routines into more of a workout. Adidas, one of my company's sponsors, even has a new 'MOVE' shoe with a pedometer built into the heel that calculates your steps throughout the day. The MOVE, due out in February 2006, features a digital readout with seven digits to count up to 9,999,999 steps. If you make it to that point, you definitely will have made your life a workout – and need new shoes!

Remember, you're a competitive athlete in the Game of Life, and that's not just when you're working out. Throughout the day, fire those glutes, keep that tummy tight and elevate the chest. Soon you'll be gliding through life like the successful person you are.

Chapter 8 Summary: Effective workouts train the body for athletic, functional movement. It's about training *movements,* not body parts. Pillar strength, the foundation of movement, consists of shoulder, core and hip stability.

Try to work these areas beyond your workout routine. Make it a daily habit to bring your shoulders back and down as if you're putting them in your back pockets. Keep your tummy tight, and fire those glutes.

CHAPTER 9

THE CORE WORKOUT: AN INTRODUCTION

Everything in a professional athlete's life is accelerated. A single play, game, season or career can be a microcosm of the Game of Life. It's about teamwork and competition. There are challenges and adjustments and, ultimately, wins and losses.

An athlete's career is especially accelerated – some attempt to stretch their careers out to the age of 35 or 40, though most end long before that. Athletes constantly try to improve their skills and have a small window of opportunity to take advantage of them. Yet no matter how well they've done this, they've accelerated the ageing process. Their bodies have been driven so hard and crashed so many times, it's as if they've been artificially aged.

This is no different from the affect long hours at work can have on the bodies of non-athletes. For most of us, competitive athletics ends in school or university. Even those who make it as professional athletes have a career lifespan of fewer than 10 years on average, which is a lot shorter than the length of the average person's working life.

Your working career will last 40 years, perhaps longer. Thankfully, you need not endure the punishment of a rugby player, the grind of marathon training or the repetitive stress a bowler's knees undergo. Yet your deterioration is no different, just more gradual and subtle. By sitting at computers all day and remaining inactive, you lose mobility. Joints begin to lock down, and over time, you develop excruciating hip and back problems.

By not taking action now, you're not only ensuring this decline, you're expediting the process – to the point that, at all of 45 years old, you may have inflicted as much damage on your body as someone who's spent a decade playing professional sports.

I have friends between the ages of 35 and 55 who say that it hurts to get in and out of a car. They avoid squatting because it hurts their knees and back. It saddens me because they've lost part of what makes them who they are. Instead of being vibrant, happy, pain-free people, they've aged long before their time.

Research into ageing suggests that while we might not be able to live decades longer by taking care of our bodies, we can dramatically improve the quality of our remaining years. That's a key part of the Core philosophy. It's not just about the length of time, it's about the *quality* of our time. This programme arrests the natural decline of ageing, helping you to master the fundamental skills you've probably forgotten. We're going to turn on those transmitters that have been shut off from spending too much time at your desk and off your feet.

It all starts with the notion of activating your core, as we discussed in the previous chapter.

You want to keep your shoulders pulled back and down and your tummy tight. You also want to initiate movement from your hips and glutes.

If you suffer from back or joint pain, haven't exercised in years and possess a lack of energy and muscle tightness, you're going to get out of the rut by using some of the same simple principles we use with world-class athletes, but don't be intimidated by that. Many of the athletes we see have the same problems you do. It's just that the stresses of their sport have expedited the process.

I want you to look at *Core Performance Essentials* as the slip road to the performance motorway. The further down we go on that motorway, the further away we are from ageing and deconditioning. It's never too early to jump on the motorway. I hope that children follow this programme, too, since they're more susceptible to premature ageing than previous generations because of a lack of activity, more screen time, and exposure to processed and fast foods. If children can master this programme, they will rank among the top 10 per cent of youth in terms of fitness. Should they want to play sport, this will put them ahead of the game, and get them ready for the highest levels of competition. Even if they don't want to play sport, they'll be on the road to a long and healthy life. Studies suggest that obese children become obese adults. The Core programme gives us a way to prevent that. There's always been a school of thought that children should avoid resistance training, since their bones are still growing. But look at how young children move: they jump off a playground slide or climb monkey bars. There are more forces on joints and musculature in those movements than we could ever create with resistance training. This workout is great for children, but like anything else, there must be a level of mastery and progression. We're not going to hand a child – or an adult – a huge weight without teaching him how to perform the movement properly using only his body weight.

Most people remain motivated to work out through the teenage and early adult years, if only because they have more time and are looking to impress potential mates. Once you factor a full-time job into the equation, it becomes more difficult, but you can still make the time.

Some people slack off from fitness once they've found a mate or started a family, but that should be only the *beginning* of a lifelong commitment to health. Now you have responsibility for someone other than yourself. Between a spouse, home ownership and perhaps children, you have even more reasons to want to ensure that you'll be around for a long time.

As the pace of life increases exponentially because of the demands of having a family – including taking care of children and, perhaps, elderly parents – life becomes more hectic. Time becomes more precious, and you need this workout solution to maintain the quality of your life.

Time is the only limiting factor. It's the downfall of many fitness programmes because there's no progression. People do the same exercises until their bodies are so used to the programme that there's no longer a benefit. In some cases, they've made matters worse by creating muscle imbalances. With *Core Performance Essentials,* the progression is unlimited. You're not going to be that person in the gym doing the same routine with the same weight at the same time year after year. The more you progress, the more movements you're able to integrate. Results increase, and in less time.

It's like the Japanese concept of *Kaizen,* which we translate as 'continuous improvement'. In the West, we tend to look for quick fixes and dramatic turnarounds, whether in business or fitness. There's nothing wrong with that mentality, but it often does not come with a foundation for long-term success.

Kaizen strives for steady, uninterrupted, incremental change. It's originally a Buddhist term meaning 'Renew the heart and make it good', and that's a literal encapsulation of exactly what we're doing. We're renewing the heart and the rest of the body by increasing its capacity, making it as good and productive as it can be.

Each day, we'll take tiny steps by increasing the amount of weight, the complexity of the movement or the number of repetitions. We can increase the challenge of balancing by going from two legs to one or by incorporating a physioball. By increasing the 'work density', we continually progress by getting more quality work done in less time.

Work density is a key component of this programme. In many bodybuilding-based exercise regimes, your work density is limited. You perform 1 set and then rest for at least that long, perhaps while spotting someone, before doing another. As a result, you learn to pace yourself. That's not the case with the Core Workout, because you're constantly moving. And as you become more proficient with the movements, you will do more in less time, thus enabling you either to add more exercises, circuits, reps or simply perform advanced versions of the ones you're already doing. Either way, you're constantly progressing with the same investment of time.

You can customize the schedule to fit your needs. If you want to work out at home with no equipment, fine. If you have limited access to equipment on the road, we'll show you what to do. Maybe you'd like to invest in a home gym to save time commuting to a gym. Instead of paying a month's gym fees, take that money and assemble your own home Core gym.

To get an idea of the type of equipment you might want to buy as you progress, visit the online shop at *www.coreperformance.com*, where we list a range of products. We've tested all of the equipment on the Web site at Athletes' Performance. You can purchase the equipment from our online shop, which can ship merchandise internationally, or use our list of equipment as a guide to what to look for in shops in your own town.

These versatile, inexpensive pieces of equipment, such as mini bands, elastic tubing home gyms, adjustable dumbbells, slideboard tops, physioballs, medicine balls and foam rolls, don't take up a large amount of space. The Core Workout is designed so that it can adapt and grow with your needs. Recognizing that there will be times when you're limited by a lack of equipment, we've provided options. Here, then, are the four units of the Core Workout.

MOVEMENT PREPARATION

Movement Preparation is an active series of warmup exercises that will efficiently increase your core temperature; lengthen, strengthen, stabilize and balance your muscles; and, as the name suggests, prepare the body for movement.

Perhaps you're accustomed to performing static, stretch-and-hold exercises that seem like a precursor to actually working out. That's not the case with Movement Prep. As with everything else in the Core Workout, you're making the most of your time. You're warming up and preparing for movement, but this is part of the actual workout. In fact, if you ever get to the end of the day and realize that you have not worked out, do the Movement Prep routine. If you're that pressed for time, you can at least make this 5-minute investment in your long-term health.

With Movement Prep, you're going to both lengthen and strengthen your muscles in the same movement. Movement Prep will help to

'I haven't felt this good since I was 9!'

NAME: MARSHALL VINER

AGE: 42

OCCUPATION: ESTATE AGENT

Marshall Viner thought his days as an active athlete were over. He spent his teenage years playing football and working in the physically taxing business of commercial fishing, straining his back to lift nets and hoist fish. At 18, he endured a horrific accident, landing on his spine.

Doctors told him he never would play sport again and that he would endure back trouble for the rest of his life. Eventually, he was diagnosed with juvenile discogenic disease, a degenerative spinal condition that causes excruciating back pain.

Through the years, Viner has endured surgeries, visited chiropractors and undergone agonizing physiotherapy. All helped, but he still could not run without pain in his hips and back.

His job as an estate agent involves lunches with clients and late dinners. Soon, he had put 86 kilograms (190 pounds) onto his 1.65-metre (5-foot-5) frame, which only exacerbated his back problems.

Then, Viner tried the Core programme and found that he could run without pain. Soon he was running 50–65 kilometres (30 to 40

miles) a week on a treadmill. He lost 9 kilograms (20 pounds).

'It feels so good to be this mobile,' Viner says. 'My back hasn't felt this good since I was 9!'

Viner finds it most effective to do some Core training after swimming or treadmill work. 'It's given me phenomenal results,' he says. 'I wish I had known about this programme 20 years ago. A lot of people suffer from back pain and figure there's nothing they can do about it. That's not the case. You've got to find a way to keep moving. This programme has shows how.'

re-establish the mobility, coordination and joint stability you enjoyed in your younger years and it's going to improve strength, balance and co-ordination – in other words, it will heighten your body's ability to process information.

This is not about developing rippling abdominal muscles to support your lower back – that's just one piece of the puzzle. Instead, you're going to perform the fundamental movements necessary to sustain and enjoy life, re-

establishing the chains that were broken as you became less active.

You want to improve the long-term mobility and flexibility of muscles. Rather than have them stretch and go back to where they were – as is the case with traditional stretch-and-hold routines – you want your body to remember these new ranges of motion.

This is done through a process of lengthening the muscle (known as active elongation), which is more effective than a traditional stretch. Here's the crucial difference: after you stretch the muscle to this new range of motion, you stabilize, then contract through the new range of motion. In other words, you don't just stretch your muscles and let them snap back into place, like a rubber band. Instead, you show your muscles how to use the motion.

I don't care how out of shape or tight you are. No matter how much your knees or back hurt, you can do the exercises listed in Level 1. There are no excuses. So many people refuse to work out because they have such ailments, and that only leads to more discomfort. By not working out, you will hurt more, and your quality of life will deteriorate. If you just follow this Movement Prep routine, however, you will eliminate the symptoms and thus your excuses for not exercising. All it takes is a desire to move better and experience less pain.

Once you've mastered Movement Prep, you will know the Core movements you need to protect your body from the long-term deterioration of ageing and overuse.

PREHAB

That brings us to the concept of what I call Prehab. You're no doubt familiar with rehabilitation, or 'rehab', which often is needed to recover from injuries brought about from a lack of movement or exercise.

With the Core Prehab routine, you're going to protect your body from backsliding into the pain, inactivity and dysfunction that lead to the downwards spiral. Prehab is a valuable insurance policy. If you do nothing else but Movement Prep and Prehab, you will maintain the physical abilities you need to lead an engaged, full, active life. (You should, however, add the Strength and Cardio units to the mix to maximize energy and long-term health.)

Wherever life takes you, Prehab is something you can do in a few minutes each day to maintain your body. This routine (see page 141) protects you from shoulder pain, lower-back trouble, hip pain and knee and foot ailments. It will give you the necessary balance, coordination, strength and endurance to function in everyday life.

Prehab, along with Movement Prep, will give you the basic requirements for all human movement, the absolute minimum to sustain quality of life. And yet, 90 per cent of people cannot perform these basic movements. Master Prehab and you'll be among the top.

Regardless of how crazy life gets, make time to do your Prehab exercises just three times a week. As long as you can perform Movement Prep and Prehab, you will be well-prepared to face middle age and your later years. You will be less likely to endure crippling back pain and hip ailments, which may cause both premature ageing and entry into a nursing home or even hospital down the road.

The lack of long-term goals is a problem in

most workout routines. They get you into shape for short-term goals, but there's no long-term vision. If you're only motivated by a school reunion, a wedding or a beach holiday, you'll be less likely to make a lasting commitment. Let those events be motivational – for what you want to look and feel like for the rest of your life.

Even pro athletes are guilty of this short-sightedness. Their careers end and they stop all activity. It's amazing how often you see a former football player hobble onto the field to be honoured before a game. Inevitably, he's put on 14 kilograms (30 pounds) and struggles just to trot out to wave to the crowd.

But at least that guy probably stayed active into his late thirties. Most people quit long before that, retiring from the Game of Life well before their prime. If only they had invested some time in Prehab.

Remember that Prehab is not a short-term solution. You will experience immediate results, to be sure, but there needs to be a long-term commitment. Nothing less than your long-term health and quality of life is at stake.

This is true of the entire Core programme: It's a progression, and if you want great results, you have to stick with it. Firstly, we stop the bad habits of poor eating and inactivity, thus decreasing your pain. That's where the Core Nutrition chapter and Movement Prep came in. Now we're going to help you become active, thus preventing future pain. And that's the beauty of Prehab: you will be investing in your long-term health and productivity, which leads to a strong performance in the Game of Life.

STRENGTH

Once we've mastered the Movement Prep and Prehab routines, we're going to add some strength training. Isn't it interesting that people always refer to *weight* training, not strength training? After all, you're training to become stronger.

Too many people lift the same weights, week after week, and year after year. Their bodies adapt and stop getting stronger. These people probably follow bodybuilding-based programmes that make no effort to work the core or to train for functional movement.

We, however, will focus on multi-joint movements that improve coordination and recruit lots of muscles, a process that expends more energy and gives more return on our investment of time. It will burn calories and improve balance, stability, flexibility, strength and the cardiovascular system all at once.

This is where you become more and more efficient. As you master these movements, you'll find that they take less time. By training in a circuit, alternating movements that emphasize different regions of the body, you will be in constant motion.

If you work out in a gym, you'll find that you will do 2 or 3 sets for every 1 set that the people around you complete, because they rest between sets. You'll keep the routine to 30 minutes, with a goal of seeing how much energy you can expend in that time frame. You will be in perpetual motion. This is the difference between flying through life with a sense of direction and meandering through life like a goalie, fending off shots.

Strength training will increase your lean body mass, which is the key to a healthy physique. After the age of 25, we lose 500 grams (1 lb) of lean body mass each year unless we do something about it. For each 500 grams (1 lb) of extra lean body mass you have, you burn an extra 50 calories a day. Even when you sleep, you'll burn more calories.

It's the difference between having a four-cylinder or an eight-cylinder engine. The eight-cylinder is going burn more fuel. Sure, it requires more fuel, but as we established in the Core Nutrition programme, a hot fire burns more fuel. You'll be eating more often and fuelling your body with nothing but the equivalent of high-octane petrol.

We've set up this programme to ease you into the circuit training programme. At the start of the programme, you won't do any strength exercises at all. You'll never do more than six exercises, all progressing at a gradual pace. Once you've experienced the benefits of Movement Prep and Prehab, you'll have the foundation to perform the Strength regime at maximum capacity. If you're pressed for time, do only Movement Prep and Prehab and find some time in your day for cardio exercise – for example, taking the stairs instead of the lift at work – and you'll be fine.

Even though the strength workout is not aerobic exercise, you will get some aerobic benefit from the workout as your heart rate will increase because of the continuous movement and will remain high throughout the workout. It's as if you're getting an aerobic workout, a two-for-one bonus. It's another example of how you will get the maximum benefit out of your 30 minutes.

By building strength and lean body mass through circuit training, you'll elevate your metabolism, and that elevated rate will last for *a few days,* as opposed to low-level cardiovascular training, which only gives the metabolism a short-term burst while exercising and in the hours immediately afterwards.

One of the goals of this programme is to increase work capacity, which is another measure of fitness. This is sometimes referred to as work density – a measure of how much work gets done per unit of time. If I gave you *X* units' worth of work and it took you 30 minutes to accomplish today, with practice, it might only take 15 minutes 3 weeks later. Thus, you can accomplish more during that 30-minute period.

Your ability to perform in Level 4 will be the best indication of your current fitness. If you ever get knocked off of your Core programme, you can figure out when you are back to your best by working back up to the level and stage you left off with, and then progressing from there.

That's a concrete way to measure increased fitness: more quality and quantity in less time. It's like fast broadband versus dial-up internet.

You can measure progress in terms of time, number of repetitions, amount of weight used and the number of times you can complete the circuit. If for some reason you miss a few workouts – or even a few weeks – you'll be able to measure the regression by discovering just how much you can get done in 30 minutes, and how it compares with your results before you fell off the programme.

Strength training in the Core programme is not just about increasing the strength of your larger muscles. It improves *stabilizing* strength, which supports proper alignment, movement patterns and energy transfer and helps to reduce injuries. In short, the Strength unit acts as a foundation for all movement. The strength exercises we've selected are designed to increase your stabilizing strength most efficiently, and after we direct you to work on one movement, we've built in enough time to allow that area to recover while you work on something else. We'll start with an exercise that's an 'upper-body push', such as press-ups or an alternating dumbbell press. From there, we'll proceed to a 'lower-body pull', then to an 'upper-body pull' and a 'lower-body push', all in a circuit fashion. We'll tie it all together with additional core work and rotational movements.

The Core Strength circuit increases the number of muscles being recruited throughout different parts of the body, to optimize your bloodflow and release positive hormones. By alternating exercises like this, you'll be able to do a few more reps each time or use a little more weight, and all in a shorter period of time. As a result, you'll increase the workout density – the quality and quantity of work per unit of time – improve your overall fitness, and enjoy cardiovascular benefits while increasing your balance, flexibility, stability and mobility.

CARDIO (A.K.A. ENERGY-SYSTEM DEVELOPMENT)

Cardio work is perhaps the most misunderstood and most debated element of fitness. Some believe that it's unnecessary and prefer to focus exclusively on resistance training. Others misinterpret cardio training as a slog, which provides little return on investment of time. Whatever the case, I'm not a big fan of the term *cardio* because it's come to represent long, slow, sloppy movement. For most people, it means going out for a jog at the same steady pace for an hour, employing poor, inefficient movement patterns. For others, it entails hopping on a stationary bike, stairclimber or treadmill for a steady but hardly strenuous 45 minutes.

This, obviously, does not provide a high return on your investment of time, and it goes against everything you're trying to accomplish with *Core Performance Essentials*. We want you to get more out of your 30 minutes on Tuesdays and Thursdays than others do who maintain a leisurely, undemanding pace.

Because of circuit training, you're already

INCREASE YOUR HORSEPOWER

In the world of thoroughbred racing, interval training is controversial. Owners of million-dollar horses do not want to risk injury by having the animals pushed through interval training. Unless the training is carefully monitored, it's possible that a horse's legs could buckle during the work interval.

Rather than take that risk, many owners prefer to rely on the horse's superior genetics and traditional training methods, which are the equine equivalent of going on a long, slow run or spending 30 leisurely minutes on a piece of gym equipment.

In many cases, that's sufficient. But there have been instances of US$10,000 horses undergoing interval training and outracing million-dollar opponents. That's not a bad metaphor for the Core Essentials programme. After all, the successful person is the one that departs from the pack to try something different, who relies not on natural gifts but on hard work and the will to constantly improve.

Unlike a thoroughbred horse, we don't have the advantage of being bred for physical performance. But by undergoing interval training, we can greatly increase our horsepower.

---

benefiting from a degree of cardio work. If you're making progress and increasing your workload, perhaps monitoring it with a pedometer, you're going to achieve an impressive cardio result. Don't feel bad if you don't have time for a dedicated cardio workout every Tuesday and Thursday, because even without it, you're going to achieve results.

But just as you're investing the 30 minutes, 3 days a week, you'll get a phenomenal return on investment if you add 30 minutes of cardio, 2 days a week in Level 1. You might find that it helps you stick with your daily workout ritual and that it enables you to expend more calories by getting your body and mind moving.

Since this programme is all about progression, I prefer to use terms such as *interval training* or Energy System Development. But

since *cardio* is so universally used, we'll stick with it here, recognizing that we're going to redefine the term.

Cardio is more than the 30 minutes you'll spend on Tuesdays and Thursdays. For starters, I want you to lead a more active lifestyle. Take the stairs instead of the lift. Instead of circling the car park for the closest spot, park in the first one that's available and walk further to the shops. Ride a bike wherever you can, even to work, if possible. Take the dog for a walk. Instead of sitting around watching your child's football practice, walk around the field a few times, keeping an eye on the action.

Look for opportunities to move and exert energy. Avoid lifts. Walk, don't ride, escalators. Walk briskly alongside those moving walkways at the airport. Otherwise, you'll probably get stuck behind someone riding the walkway. (And there's that obesity epidemic again!) Life is one big workout. Take advantage of the dozens of opportunities in front of you every day.

In Levels 2, 3 and 4, you'll be ready to take 1 of the 2 days and mix in some light 'intervals' – periods of moderate exercise alternated with intense periods. With intervals, there will be times when I want you to work harder. Drop the conversation with your friends in the gym for a few moments, focus on working harder, and your heart rate will elevate. If you're out walking, try a light jog for 30 seconds to a couple of minutes, and then slow once more to a walk. Try to incorporate four to eight intervals during the course of your half-hour walk.

Intensity is far more important than volume. You're going to maintain the same volume – 12 to 30 minutes – throughout the programme, but you'll ratchet up the intensity as you go along.

The smaller the ratio of work to rest, the more you will improve your body's *lactate threshold* – its capacity to do high-intensity work. With anaerobic exercise, which is exercise done at maximum effort, the body relies more on energy stores than it does on oxygen. It puts you in oxygen debt, which increases the burning sensation in muscles and makes the body compensate to get your heart rate to come back down.

But there's tremendous benefit to this. It's like a tuning a high-performance engine – in this case, the lungs, heart and related systems. Interval training increases energy production in every cell and in the connections to those cells, allowing you to burn energy more efficiently.

With most cardio work, people believe that they're exercising much harder than they really are. Some gyms have 'perceived exertion charts' on the wall where people can attach a number figure to how they feel. Most people go by sweat, which often is a function of how long they've been on the machine (if not the temperature in the room) and not how hard they've been working.

Gym equipment provides an effective cardio workout. Jump aboard a bike, treadmill, elliptical trainer or stepping machine. Set it on manual. Many of these machines are equipped with heart rate monitors. You grasp the handles, and within seconds the machine gives you a reading. But just because they're appropriate for the task, don't feel limited to gym machines. (Heart rate monitors are inexpensive tools and can be bought in most sports shops.) If you'd rather do your cardio work by attacking hills, cycling or even swimming, then by all means go for it. You could climb stairs or run a daunting hill in your neighbourhood. Maybe there's a route that has a series of hills and flat surfaces. Wherever you choose to do your Cardio work, by following the *Core Performance Essentials* Workout you'll enjoy a cardio benefit, although it's important to do something else. Be active throughout the day and try to get in your 30 minutes of cardio.

It's never too early or too late to start. According to a number of recent studies, cardio-respiratory fitness in early adulthood can significantly decrease the chance of developing high blood pressure and diabetes, which are both major risk factors for heart disease and stroke in later life.

That's no surprise, of course. But the key is to maximize your effort with proper movement patterns through cardio work, not just to make the most of your time but also to safeguard your health, now and for the future.

The Cardio routine evolves in each of the four levels and stages. Each one starts with a warmup period of 3 minutes and a cooldown period ranging from 3 to 5 minutes, which will take you up to 30 minutes for each workout.

Cardio is no time to get sloppy with movement patterns. Regardless of the activity, you should feel tall and stabilized through your pillar. Focus on keeping both feet pointing straight ahead. Fire your glutes and quads, and don't forget to use your arms. You will be amazed at how much more fluid you feel, and at the amount of speed you can maintain with less effort.

In Level 1, we will focus on steady-state aerobic work. *Aerobic* simply means that your body will use oxygen to provide a steady and consistent, low level of energy for a long time, without building up any waste products in the body that hinder performance.

Think of it as a low-horsepower, highly fuel-efficient, four-cylinder engine that can run all day but does not generate a whole lot of power. A good rule of thumb for Level 1 is that you should be able to carry on a conversation when you are in the aerobic zone.

Some of the best activities for Level 1 are:

- Outdoors: brisk walking, walking up hills, cycling, swimming, rowing
- Indoors on cardio equipment: cycling, treadmill climbing/walking, elliptical trainer

Using the aerobic zone during Level 1 will improve your cardiovascular system and prepare your muscles for the greater speeds of Levels 2 through 4. This lower-level work will let your movement patterns, muscles and joints adapt and prepare for the more intense training coming in these next phases.

When we get into Levels 2, 3 and 4, we will introduce interval training, where there will be bouts of harder effort mixed with easier-effort periods to give your body time to recover. We will use the lower-intensity Level 1 aerobic work in Levels 2 through 4 – the more advanced zones of the programme – as the recovery tool.

As with the Core Strength unit, interval training increases your body's release of positive hormones, which builds lean body mass and signals your body to dump fat. At the same time, it keeps your heart rate from dropping out of the aerobic zone.

Level 2 will introduce interval training by mixing moderate intensity work with bouts of Level 1 easy-intensity aerobic work to allow you to catch your breath and recover from the slightly more intense intervals.

You will notice that these exercises include some work and some rest; we call this the work-to-rest ratio. The greater the rest, the higher quality the work should be. The lower the ratio – for instance, 1 second of rest per 1 second of work (one-to-one) – the bigger the challenge will be, since the body has less time to recover. That will increase your capacity to do more work.

You'll know you've reached Level 2 moderate intensity if you would find it difficult to carry on a conversation. You could talk, but you wouldn't be able to say much more than a couple of words at a time.

Some of the best activities for Level 2 are:

● Outdoors: running-to-jogging/walking, jogging-to-walking

● Indoors: cycling, elliptical trainer, treadmill, stairclimbers

In Level 3, you will work harder. We are going to decrease the times and increase the rest intervals. Don't be intimidated by more intense work; you'll be ready for it. In fact, you will be looking for a greater challenge.

That brings us to Level 4, the shortest of the intervals. It's going to require you to use all of this newfound mobility, stability and strength. At this level you will run, ride or climb as hard as possible for between 10 and 30 seconds. In order to get the most out of Level 4, you'll need to pack as much power and energy into these segments as possible.

Some of the best activities for Level 4 are:

● Sprinting (flat or uphill)

● Shuttle runs (5 metres and back, 10 metres and back, 15 metres and back)

● Bicycle intervals

● Stairclimber or stepping machine sprints

The bottom line with the Core Cardio unit is that instead of slow, plodding workouts, we want to create a process where your muscles, nervous system and hormones act together in efficient movement patterns that help your body to work as efficiently as possible.

Chapter 9 Summary: The Core Workout is an integrated programme that trains the body for lifelong movement. It consists of four components: Movement Preparation, Prehab, Strength and Cardio. Movement Prep increases core temperature and lengthens and strengthens muscles so that you make long-term flexibility and stability gains. Prehab is the proactive approach to protecting yourself from injury by building 'pillar strength', the integration of shoulder, trunk and hip stability. Your body needs strength to sustain movement and everyday demands. We will improve the strength of the movements you were born with. Unlike traditional cardio work, the Core Cardio unit focuses on quality, not quantity, and it improves the function of your cardiovascular system while building endurance and helping your body to create new energy levels.

CHAPTER 10

CORE MOVEMENTS

I n 2005, the US Department of Health and Human Services issued new guidelines to combat the nation's growing weight problem. Other countries have issued similar guidelines. Adults should do about 60 minutes of 'moderate to vigorous' physical activity daily to prevent weight gain. Those trying to maintain weight loss should do 60 to 90 minutes. Previous guidelines called for just 30 minutes a day – and just one-third of adults reached that goal. So I'm guessing that with the bar raised, the percentages will get even worse. The problem with these recommendations is that they assume people work out at a meandering pace, if at all, and never push themselves.

All I want you to start with is exercise 3 days a week (Monday, Wednesday and Friday) for 30 minutes at a time. If you have time to do some cardio work on Tuesdays and Thursdays, then that's great – try to make the most of those additional 30-minute intervals.

Anyone can find 30 minutes, 3 days a week, to make this small investment in his life. That's just 1.3 per cent of your waking hours, assuming 8 hours of sleep a night. If you can make that commitment, I guarantee that the return on your investment will be exponential.

No matter how busy you are, you can find 30 minutes. Turn off the television – or at least set the VCR. Get up earlier. Instead of going out to lunch, take advantage of that health club in your office. Schedule your workouts on a day planner or BlackBerry. That way, they'll become a core component of your lifestyle.

The upside is tremendous. Not only will you feel and look better, but you'll also create a body that's resistant to injury, long-term deterioration and excruciating back pain. By following this programme, in conjunction with the Core Nutrition guidelines, you will build long-term health, not just temporary muscles.

Isn't it amazing that people take better care of their cars than of their bodies? They pay for oil changes and services. They rotate the tyres and change all of the filters and belts, all with the hope of getting maximum performance and the longest possible lifespan out of a vehicle unlikely to last more than 10 years, no matter how well they take care of it.

Why not take the same approach with your body? After all, you can always buy a new car, but your body you can't replace. Money and extended warranties can cure most automotive problems. That's not the case with your health.

Speaking of money, think of how diligent people are when it comes to preparing financially for middle age and retirement: they make short-term sacrifices in order to properly finance university funds for their children, retirement accounts and other investments so that they can enjoy their golden years in comfort.

But what good is financial security if you're sick or confined to a wheelchair during your retirement? What good is financial security if you're lost to a stroke or heart attack? Taking just 90 minutes a week is a far smaller sacrifice than the ones you're probably already making for your financial future. Unlike financial planning, with its degree of uncertainty and risk, you know you'll get a return from this investment. Make this modest investment now and you can remain active well into your seventies, eighties and nineties, improving the quality of your life.

With this programme, we've eliminated all excuses. If you can't make it to a gym, we've provided exercise variations that can be done with nothing more than a mini band, a physioball and a pair of dumbbells at home. If you're on the road or have no access to equipment, we've included versions that require nothing at all.

But wait, you say, it will take some time to get up to speed with the programme. You've never done anything like this before. If that's the case, stop after 30 minutes. That's right. Call it a day. Pat yourself on the back. You'll find that as you master the movements, you can do the workout faster and thus get through more of it.

Our goal is not to create longer workouts but to pack more into our limited time. If you are already working out, you will have to think of your routines differently. You're not going to rest between sets or alternate exercises with a partner. Instead, you'll train opposite sets of movements, which is to say movements that tax different muscle groups, in circuits so that you don't need to stop. Work with your partner at the same time. By maintaining this pace, you'll find that the Movement Prep, Prehab and Strength elements of *Core Performance Essentials* form a cardio workout in themselves.

Since you're no doubt accustomed to multi-tasking in other areas of life, this should not be too much of an adjustment. Don't confuse this with talking on the mobile phone or conducting business while working out. That's counterproductive – and disrespectful to the people you're talking to and those around you at the gym. Make this time for yourself.

If you think this workout is too easy, add sets, reps or exercises to the Core Workout. Perform the advanced routines. Your progress is unlimited, though time is not. If you haven't tried the workouts in my first book, *Core Performance,* you might want to give them a shot.

The reason most people spend so much time in the gym – or think that it's necessary – is because they never improve their work density. They add more reps, sets and exercises, but because they work at a slow, plodding pace, it takes more time. We're not going to do that.

Have you ever prepared to give a speech or talk? If so, you've probably noticed that the more you practise, the shorter the talk becomes. It's not necessarily because you're talking faster or truncating parts, but you're becoming more comfortable with what you're saying. You might find that you can pack more into that 30-minute talk than you thought.

That's the same philosophy as with this workout. As you get more comfortable, you work more efficiently.

I've divided the Core Workout into four levels, which fall into three colour zones: Red, Yellow and Green. Think of it as a traffic light. Red means *stopping* your *inactivity.* If your body is tight, in pain or out of shape, that's going to stop right here. You fall into the Red category if:

● You're really out of shape, meaning you haven't worked out in years – or ever.

● You're coming off an injury-related layoff.

● You get some exercise, but your body is very tight – for instance, if you can't remember the last time you touched your toes.

● You used to work out regularly but, because of added time constraints and new responsibilities, you haven't been doing much exercise in recent months or years.

As with a traffic light, you should use caution in the Yellow Zone. You've loosened up your body and have made progress in the Red Zone, but you're not quite ready for the Green Zone.

Marketing – 'no pain, no gain' – has taught us that if we want to look like bodybuilders or fitness or fashion models, we must undergo daily suffering. When we don't achieve those results, despite Herculean efforts, we feel inadequate and disappointed. Workout programmes fail not because people lack commitment but because they grind themselves down by doing more kilometres or repetitions than they need until they have punished their bodies into submission.

Instead of falling into that pattern, stop while you're ahead. That way, when you come back for more, you'll be ready to achieve an even higher level of performance. Don't get me wrong; this programme will help you to look noticeably different in 3 short weeks. But you'll accomplish it the right way, with a view to the long run, to make sure you feel and perform better. The bottom line is that we need to shift our mindsets by understanding this new paradigm with these three main goals:

1. Decreasing pain (Red Zone – Level 1)

2. Preventing pain (Yellow Zone – Level 2)

3. Performing (Green Zone – Levels 3 and 4)

This traffic light analogy applies to training and to many other aspects of life. Before we are able to move forwards in terms of our bodies, relationships or finances, we must stop the downwards spiral. We must decrease physical pain to enjoy the quality of life we deserve.

Once the pain is diminished, we're free to exercise with the intent of regaining that lost function and 'prehab' to make sure it does not happen again.

Think of this as building the agility to quickly change directions in life. This is the line in the sand where you stop going in the wrong direction. Take a rugby player going forward as an analogy. He is heading one way, then he stops and explodes in another direction, sprinting for his goal of scoring again, but always moving forwards, and never backwards.

It takes less-conditioned athletes longer to do this; some would call them slow. Highly conditioned athletes do it almost instantaneously, all game long. To be great athletes in the Game of Life, we have to do this several times per hour, as the tacklers (stress and chaos) force us to redirect ourselves and immediately continue on towards our core values and goals.

The Core Workout is organized into four levels or 'zones':

Level 1

The Red Zone, also known as Level 1 of the Core Workout, will be the springboard to your success in the Game of Life.

You're in the Red Zone because of pain that's keeping you from leading the quality of life you deserve. You have less energy and motivation to exercise, since it causes more pain. It is a degenerating and depressing free fall.

We all go through this pain at some point in

our lives if we don't take preventive action. Maybe you're there already. We don't know what the Game of Life will throw at us, but we can take action now to prevent the decline. It all starts with getting out of the Red Zone and heading for the motorway of life.

Level 2

When you see a yellow light, you think 'caution'. Maybe you floor the accelerator and speed through the light, or perhaps you come to a stop. It depends mostly on your position at the moment.

In our Yellow Zone, Level 2, we're exercising caution to make sure that we prevent injuries down the road. We can actually prevent more than 65 per cent of injuries in sport and everyday life. We also can do a better job of preparing for and protecting ourselves from the severity of the remaining 35 per cent of injuries, which are caused by traumatic events and accidents.

In the Yellow Zone of the Core Workout, we will focus on how to protect the most vulnerable areas of the body, making sure that everything is aligned and working in harmony. That way, there will be no excessive wear and tear caused by poor movement patterns. An ounce of prevention goes a very long way in life.

Levels 3 and 4

Now that you have taken the time to restore your body and protect it from injury, you will feel the desire to use it. By applying this energy in the right ways, you will fly down the performance motorway.

As you enter the motorway, you have to pick a slip road and start building up speed towards your destination, and that's exactly what you will do here. As you master and progress through Levels 3 and 4 of the Core Performance Essentials system, you will be able to merge with other high-performance vehicles through my first book, *Core Performance,* or better yet, through a version that's customized for you at *www.coreperformance.com*.

You will never be overly challenged, nor will you ever be bored to death and stifled by doing the same old thing. Being part of the Core community ensures your progress and evolution with convenient, fun and affordable alternatives.

The Core Movement programme will use these three goals – decreasing pain (Level 1, the Red Zone), preventing pain (Level 2, the Yellow Zone) and performing (Levels 3 and 4, the Green Zone) – from the very first Level 1 programme to the highest levels of performance that the most elite athletes achieve during their career.

Now let's take a look at how we're going to progress through the exercises. Firstly, I want you to achieve and experience some success. After that, I will be honoured to gradually challenge you more and more until you look back one day and shake your head in disbelief over how far you have come.

Let's begin by aiming for just 30 minutes of exercise three times a week and focus on achieving the highest return on your time investment. We will fire up this engine, and it will take on a life of its own because it will become part of *your* core.

In chapter 12, Quality of Time, you will be asked to block out a consistent 30 minutes a day, three times a week for your Core Routine, with a day in between for simple cardio and regeneration, which may be done all at once or throughout the day. (See chapter 11 for more on the concept of Regeneration.)

We have created a simple, progressive, four-level programme that will keep you challenged for years to come.

You will begin each level with Stage A, requiring 1 set of 6 repetitions, building up to where you can go through part of this workout twice. As soon as you are able to perform these exercises properly in the allotted time, you will add 2 reps, for a total of 8. You will then repeat this process, and bump up by 2 more reps, to 10 reps.

When you can go through the levels for the prescribed number of circuits per unit (Movement Prep, Prehab, Strength), and the desired number of reps with movement mastery, do something special for yourself. Compare notes with fellow Core participants. Celebrate victories in life and share them with your family and friends. You are then ready to move up to the next level.

The next level will repeat the same process, but I have added an exercise to each unit and increased the complexity. I will increase the demands ever so slightly within each unit and each exercise by increasing

LEVEL	STAGE A	STAGE B	STAGE C	STAGE D	TIME DISTRIBUTION
1	1×6	2×6	2×8	2×10	Movement Prep: 15 min Prehab: 15 min
2	1×6	2×6	2×8	2×10	Movement Prep: 10 min Prehab: 10 min Strength: 10 min
3	1×6	2×6	2×8	2×10	Movement Prep: 7 min Prehab: 8 min Strength: 15 min
4	1×6	2×6	2×8	2×10	Movement Prep: 7 min Prehab: 8 min Strength: 15 min

the range of motion or stability, mobility, balance or strength required. Or I might have decreased the amount of time allotted to complete the unit.

LEVEL 1: THE RED ZONE

Everyone starts here, with a 30-minute commitment, three times in Week One. Consider it your birth, indoctrination or pre-game warmup for the Core Routine. We're all newcomers to the Core Routine, and just like every newcomer in every other sport, we too have to show up to training camp before the veterans. Even if you've done the *Core Performance* routine in the past, this will be a good refresher.

This runs parallel to the nutrition chapter, where we started by eating four healthy meals, 4 days a week. Here we will learn four exercises in Movement Prep and four exercises in Prehab. The goal of this workout is to take an inventory of your body – right side versus left, front versus back, areas of tightness, balance, coordination and strength. Next, you should perfect these movements and gain confidence by awakening all those long-dormant little muscles.

How long you stay at this level depends on several factors. If you are in fairly good shape and progressing easily, you might need only 1 week before moving on to Level 2. For example, you might do Stage A and find that you have plenty of time on the clock to do one more round of each unit, which is Stage B.

That may very well mean that you're ready to graduate to Stage C on Wednesday. Here you will add 2 reps to each exercise for 2 circuits each. On Friday, you will add 2 more reps for a total of 10 repetitions in Stage D. The following week, you will start on Level 2, Stage A, and you'll find out more about what's at your core.

If you're in pain or 'deconditioned' – that is, if you're so tight that you haven't touched your toes since childhood, you have never trained before, or you've gone a long time since exercising – it might take 2 weeks to achieve mastery. Don't be alarmed if it takes longer than that. This will require patience, but think of it as turning on a car. When a car has been sitting in the garage, it takes more effort to get it started the first time. But once you do, it will come back to life quickly. Your body, likewise, will progress more rapidly from this point.

LEVEL 2: THE YELLOW ZONE

You now know the basics of the routine, but here I have added a few levels to each exercise and made the Movement Prep and Prehab routines more complex, while decreasing the time to 10 minutes for each unit. I have also added a third unit: Strength. You now have three units of five exercises, with 10 minutes to complete each unit.

In Level 2, you have to start slow and

gradually build up speed and proficiency. To make sure that you achieve gains in strength, flexibility and stability from the very first workout, you will go through each exercise unit only once, for a total of 1 set of 6 repetitions per exercise.

The goal is to formally start your training process. Here you are working on rehabbing to alleviate the discomfort you already feel and prehabbing to prevent future pain and dysfunction. This Level 2 workout will be your benchmark. If for whatever reason you get knocked off your Core Routine, you will have the resiliency of that Super Ball and bounce back quickly; you will start again with Level 2, Stage A. You will then start working up the ladder with a progressive workout that evolves each session until you face an exciting and challenging routine. This will be the baseline for your future workouts.

Remember that you have only 30 minutes, divided equally into three 10-minute blocks. Keep an eye on the clock, and get as much done as you can in one unit. If you have gone through 1½ times, and the timer goes off, stop; and move on to the next section. This is part of your challenge, decreasing your rest intervals and increasing the reps as you become more fit over time.

You will graduate from this level when you complete Stage D for 2 circuits, doing 10 perfect repetitions each, within 30 minutes.

LEVEL 3:
THE GREEN ZONE

Green means go, just as it does at the traffic lights. You are starting to get in shape. Now that you're really on the road to increased performance, let's take things up a notch.

The theme here is 'getting superstable'. I am going to challenge you in Movement Prep, first by adding another exercise, but also by having you start covering ground with every rep, which will require more balance, stability, mobility and strength.

In Prehab, there's another new exercise, taking you up to six. We'll also increase the complexity of your stabilizing strength with more 'rotary' stability, working those ever-important rotator cuffs.

The Strength circuit is also cranked up a notch by incorporating the physioball to increase the stability challenge. This will result in increased muscle recruitment and total body integration. The goal is to minimize ball movement. You might notice your body and the ball shaking – your body is trying to gain neuromuscular control by firing more often to control the unstable surface. I like to call this wasted movement and energy 'noise'. Your aim, then, is to become more efficient and silence the 'noise' by improving your ability to stabilize your body and keep the ball still.

If you need the company of others for motivation, have your training partner – whether they're with you or across the country and available only via phone or email – set the date, and go head-to-head to motivate and help each other reach new heights.

You'll note that you barely need dumbbells in Level 3. That's by design. Our goal with this unit is to stabilize our bodies, and we can do that with minimal weights. Not only that, but sometimes you're travelling or don't have access to weights for other reasons and so need a no-equipment regime.

LEVEL 4

In Level 4, we take things up yet another notch, with dumbbells to build strength. We're still in the Green Zone, only now we're going to challenge our bodies further. There might be times when you won't have access to dumbbells. When that's the case, stick with Level 3 and return to level 4 when you can access equipment.

Chapter 10 Summary: In just 30 minutes a day, you're going to change your body and your mindset about working out. You'll do this by achieving three goals: decreasing pain, preventing pain and performing at a high level. You'll progress through three workout zones: Red, Yellow and Green. As you advance, the idea is not to spend more time working out but to make the most of that 30 minutes, creating greater 'work density'. Unlike other workout regimes, the Core Workout features unlimited progressions and room for growth.

LEVEL 1: GET READY

MOVEMENT PREP
(15 MINUTES)

STAGE:	A	B	C	D
NO. OF CIRCUITS:	1	2	2	2
REPETITIONS:	6 EA	6 EA	8 EA	10 EA

1 **90/90 STRETCH**

2 **LUNGE STRETCH**

STAGE:	A	B	C	D
NO. OF CIRCUITS:	1	2	2	2
REPETITIONS:	6 EA	6 EA	8 EA	10 EA
OR TIME:	12 SEC	12 SEC	16 SEC	20 SEC

1 **TIME** **PILLAR BRIDGE FRONT** (KNEELING)

2 **REPS** **PILLAR BRIDGE LATERAL** (KNEELING)

ACTIVITIES INCLUDING: walking/jogging, cycling, swimming;
also, cardio equipment such as treadmill, stationary bike or elliptical trainer.

STAGE:	A	B	C	D
WORK: (STEADY, LOW INTENSITY)	18 MIN	18 MIN	24 MIN	30 MIN

3   **INVERTED HAMSTRING** (IN PLACE)

4   **LATERAL LUNGE**

3
TIME   **GLUTE BRIDGE** (MINI BAND)

4
REPS   **FLOOR** YS & TS

- Progress to the next <u>stage</u> when you successfully complete the prescribed number of circuits in the allotted time.

- Progress to the next <u>level</u> when you successfully complete Stage D with perfect technique in the desired time.

LEVEL 2:GET SET...GO!

MOVEMENT PREP (10 MINUTES)

STAGE:	A	B	C	D
NO. OF CIRCUITS:	1	1	1	1
REPETITIONS:	6 EA	6 EA	8 EA	10 EA

1 90/90 STRETCH (LEGS CROSSED)

2 LUNGE STRETCH (BACKWARDS)

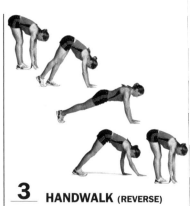

3 HANDWALK (REVERSE)

STAGE:	A	B	C	D
NO. OF CIRCUITS:	1	2	2	2
REPETITIONS:	6 EA	6 EA	8 EA	10 EA
OR TIME:	12 SEC	12 SEC	16 SEC	20 SEC

1 TIME PILLAR BRIDGE FRONT

2 TIME PILLAR BRIDGE LATERAL

3 REPS GLUTE BRIDGE (PADDED)

STRENGTH CIRCUIT (10 MINUTES)

STAGE:	A	B	C	D
NO. OF CIRCUITS:	1	2	2	2
REPETITIONS:	6 EA	6 EA	8 EA	10 EA

1 PRESS-UP (KNEELING), OR PRESS-UP

2 GLUTE BRIDGE (WITH PHYSIOBALL)

3 FLOOR CRUNCH (DOUBLE THE NUMBER OF REPS)

ACTIVITIES INCLUDING: walking/jogging, cycling, swimming; also, cardio equipment such as treadmill, stationary bike or elliptical trainer.

WARMUP: 3 MINUTES				
STAGE:	A	B	C	D
WORK: (MODERATE)	1 MIN	1 MIN	2 MIN	3 MIN
RECOVERY: (EASY)	3 MIN	3 MIN	3 MIN	3 MIN
NO. OF REPS:	3X	4X	4X	3X
COOLDOWN: 5 MINUTES				
TOTAL TIME:	20 MIN	24 MIN	28 MIN	26 MIN

4 **INVERTED HAMSTRING**
(IN PLACE)

5 **LATERAL LUNGE**
(STEP AND RETURN)

4
REPS **MINI BAND STANDING**

5
REPS **PHYSIOBALL** YS & TS
(ARMS BENT)

4 **SQUAT** (BODY WEIGHT,
WITH MINI BAND)

5 **SPLIT DUMBBELL CURL**

● Progress to the next <u>stage</u> when you successfully complete
   the prescribed number of circuits in the allotted time.

● Progress to the next <u>level</u> when you successfully complete
   Stage D with perfect technique in the desired time.

LEVEL 3: GET STABLE

MOVEMENT PREP (7 MINUTES)

STAGE:	A	B	C	D
NO. OF CIRCUITS:	1	1	1	1
REPETITIONS:	3 EA	3 EA	4 EA	5 EA

1 HIP CROSSOVER

2 LUNGE STRETCH (MOVING)

3 HANDWALK

(7 MINUTES)

STAGE:	A	B	C	D
NO. OF CIRCUITS:	1	1	1	1
REPETITIONS:	6 EA	6 EA	8 EA	10 EA
OR TIME:	12 SEC	12 SEC	16 SEC	20 SEC

1 REPS SUMO SQUAT TO HAMSTRING STRETCH

2 REPS PILLAR BRIDGE FRONT (WIDE FEET)

3 TIME PILLAR BRIDGE LATERAL (STACKED FEET)

STRENGTH CIRCUIT (15 MINUTES)

STAGE:	A	B	C	D
NO. OF CIRCUITS:	1	2	2	2
REPETITIONS:	6 EA	6 EA	8 EA	10 EA

1 PRESS-UP (WITH PHYSIOBALL)

2 GLUTE BRIDGE (WITH PHYSIOBALL LEG CURL)

3 PHYSIOBALL CRUNCH (DOUBLE THE NUMBER OF REPS)

ACTIVITIES INCLUDING: walking/jogging, cycling, swimming; also, cardio equipment such as treadmill, stationary bike, elliptical trainer or stepping machine.

	A	B	C	D
WARMUP: 3 MINUTES				
STAGE:	A	B	C	D
WORK: (HARD)	2 MIN	2 MIN	1 MIN	30 SEC
RECOVERY: (EASY)	2 MIN	2 MIN	1 MIN	30 SEC
NO. OF REPS:	3X	4X	6X	8X
COOLDOWN: 5 MINUTES				
TOTAL TIME:	20 MIN	24 MIN	20 MIN	16 MIN

4 **INVERTED HAMSTRING** (BACKWARDS)

5 **LATERAL LUNGE** (MOVING)

6 **DROP LUNGE**

4 REPS **GLUTE BRIDGE** (MARCHING)

5 REPS **MINI BAND WALKING**

6 REPS **PHYSIOBALL *Y*S & *T*S** (ARMS EXTENDED)

4 **SQUAT** (SINGLE LEG)

5 **STANDING LIFT**

6 **SPLIT DUMBBELL CURL TO PRESS**

● Progress to the next <u>stage</u> when you successfully complete the prescribed number of circuits in the allotted time.

● Progress to the next <u>level</u> when you successfully complete Stage D with perfect technique in the desired time.

LEVEL 4: GET STRONG

MOVEMENT PREP (7 MINUTES)

STAGE:	A	B	C	D
NO. OF CIRCUITS:	1	1	1	1
REPETITIONS:	5 EA	5 EA	4 EA	3 EA

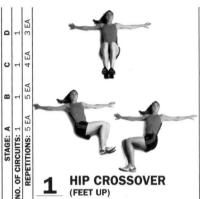

1 HIP CROSSOVER (FEET UP)

2 LUNGE STRETCH (MOVING)

3 HANDWALK

(blank middle band)

STAGE:	A	B	C	D
NO. OF CIRCUITS:	1	1	1	1
REPETITIONS:	6 EA	6 EA	8 EA	10 EA

1 PHYSIOBALL PLATE CRUNCH (DOUBLE THE NUMBER OF REPS)

2 PILLAR BRIDGE FRONT (NARROW FEET)

3 PILLAR BRIDGE LATERAL (JUMPING JACK)

STRENGTH CIRCUIT (15 MINUTES)

STAGE:	A	B	C	D
NO. OF CIRCUITS:	1	2	2	2
REPETITIONS:	6 EA	6 EA	8 EA	10 EA

1 ALTERNATING DUMBBELL BENCH PRESS

2 ROMANIAN DEADLIFT (TWO ARMS, ONE LEG)

3 ONE-ARM, ONE-LEG DUMBBELL ROW

ACTIVITIES INCLUDING: walking/sprinting, cycling, swimming; also, cardio equipment such as treadmill, stationary bike or stepping machine.

WARMUP: 3 MINUTES EASY CARDIO AND 3 MINUTES MOVEMENT PREP				
STAGE:	A	B	C	D
WORK: (VERY HARD)	10 SEC	15 SEC	20 SEC	30 SEC
RECOVERY: (EASY)	50 SEC	45 SEC	40 SEC	30 SEC
NO. OF REPS:	12X	12X	12X	12X
COOLDOWN: 5 MINUTES – MAKE SURE TO REGENERATE TONIGHT!				
TOTAL TIME:	23 MIN	23 MIN	23 MIN	23 MIN

4 **INVERTED HAMSTRING** (BACKWARD)

5 **LATERAL LUNGE** (MOVING)

6 **DROP LUNGE**

4 **GLUTE BRIDGE** (KNEE BENT)

5 **MINI BAND WALKING** (ADD RESISTANCE)

6 **PHYSIOBALL Ys & Ts** (WITH WEIGHT)

4 **SPLIT SQUAT**

5 **STANDING LIFT** (ONE LEG)

6 **ALTERNATING SPLIT DUMBBELL CURL TO PRESS**

● Progress to the next <u>stage</u> when you successfully complete the prescribed number of circuits in the allotted time.

● CONGRATULATIONS! Now progress to the next level by customizing your programme at *www.coreperformance.com*.

90/90 STRETCH

PROCEDURE:

Lie on the ground on your left side in a foetal position, with your legs tucked up into your torso at a 90-degree angle and a pad or rolled-up towel between your knees. Keep both arms straight at a 90-degree angle to your torso. Now, keeping your knees together and on the ground and your hips still, rotate your chest and right arm back to the right, trying to put your back on the ground. Exhale and hold for 2 seconds, then return to the starting position. Finish your reps, then switch sides and repeat the movement.

COACHING KEY:

Keep your knees together and pressed against the ground. Only rotate as far as you can without lifting or separating your knees. Exhale as you stretch.

YOU SHOULD FEEL:

A stretch through your torso and the muscles of your middle and upper back.

90/90 STRETCH (LEGS CROSSED)

PROCEDURE:

Lie face up on the ground holding a pad or towel roll, your left knee bent to 90 degrees, and your right leg crossed over the left. Roll over onto your left side and pin a pad between your right knee and the ground. Maintaining pressure on the pad and keeping your hips still, rotate your chest and right arm back to the right, trying to put your back on the ground. Hold for 2 seconds, then return to the starting position. Repeat until you've completed your reps, then switch sides.

MOVEMENT PREP

HIP CROSSOVER

PROCEDURE:

Lie face up on the ground with your arms to your sides, your knees bent and your feet flat. Twist your bent legs to the left until they reach the floor, then twist them to the right. Continue for the prescribed number of repetitions.

COACHING KEY:

Keep your shoulders on the ground, your knees together and your stomach tight. Do not let your knees touch the ground on either side.

YOU SHOULD FEEL:

A lengthening and strengthening of the torso.

HIP CROSSOVER (FEET UP)

Try this move with your hips and knees bent to 90 degrees and your feet off the ground. Once you master that, perform this move with your legs straight.

MOVEMENT PREP

LUNGE STRETCH

PROCEDURE:

Take a half-step forwards with your left foot, placing your right hand on the floor for balance. Take your left elbow and reach down the inside of your forward leg until you feel a stretch. Then place your left hand on the floor and push your hips upwards as you straighten your front leg. Return to the starting position and repeat.

COACHING KEY:

Contract (squeeze) the glute muscle of your back leg.

YOU SHOULD FEEL:

A stretch through the groin, the hip flexor muscle of your back leg, and the glute muscle and the hamstring of your front leg.

LUNGE STRETCH (BACKWARD)

PROCEDURE:

With your feet together, step back with your right leg into a lunge. While reaching your right hand to the sky, bend your torso to the left. Straighten your torso and step forwards into the starting position. Alternate sides and repeat for the prescribed repetitions.

MOVEMENT PREP

LUNGE STRETCH (MOVING)

PROCEDURE:

Instead of returning to the starting position as in Level 2, walk forwards into the next position.

INVERTED HAMSTRING (IN PLACE)

PROCEDURE:

Stand on one leg with perfect posture, holding on to a wall, chair or table with one hand for stability and reaching out to your side with the other hand. Keep your shoulder blades back and down. Maintaining a straight line from ear to ankle, bend over at the waist, raising your opposite heel to the sky. When you feel a stretch, return to the standing position by contracting the muscles of your hamstring, glutes and back. Complete your reps on that side, then switch legs.

COACHING KEY:

Keep your back flat and your hips and shoulders parallel to the ground. Maintain a straight line from your ear through your hip, knee and ankle. Try to keep your balance without relying on your hand, and keep your opposite foot off the ground.

YOU SHOULD FEEL:

A stretch in your hamstrings.

CORE MOVEMENTS

LEVEL 3&4

INVERTED HAMSTRING (BACKWARDS)

PROCEDURE:

Complete one rep of the movement (without a chair for support), then step back into the next step and repeat using the opposite leg, alternating legs until you've completed all your reps.

MOVEMENT PREP

LATERAL LUNGE

PROCEDURE:

Standing with your feet wider than shoulder width apart, shift your hips to the left and down by bending your left knee and keeping your right leg straight. Your feet should be straight ahead and flat on the ground. Push through your left hip, returning to the starting position. Alternate sides and then repeat.

COACHING KEY:

Keep the knee on your 'working' side behind your toes. Keep your opposite leg straight, your back flat and your chest up.

YOU SHOULD FEEL:

A lengthening and strengthening of your glutes, groin, hamstrings and your quadriceps.

LATERAL LUNGE (STEP AND RETURN)

PROCEDURE:

Step to the right with your right foot, keeping your toes forwards and your feet flat. Squat through your right hip while keeping your left leg straight. Squat as low as possible, holding this position for 2 seconds. Push back to the starting position and repeat to the opposite side.

LATERAL LUNGE (MOVING)

PROCEDURE:

Instead of returning to the starting position, step into a squat position and then into the next lunge. Repeat for the prescribed number of repetitions and then switch sides. You will be stepping around the room during this exercise, so give yourself plenty of space.

MOVEMENT PREP

HANDWALK (REVERSE)

PROCEDURE:

Bend at the waist and walk your feet out into a press-up position. Now, keeping your knees straight, walk your hands towards your feet. When you feel a stretch, walk your feet back out to a press-up position. Repeat until you've completed your reps.

COACHING KEY:

Keep your knees straight and your stomach tight. Walk your hands out further beyond your head for increased difficulty. Use short 'ankle steps' to walk back up to your hands. That is, take baby steps using only your ankles – don't use your knees, hips or quads.

YOU SHOULD FEEL:

A stretch in your hamstrings, lower back, glutes and calves.

HANDWALK

PROCEDURE:

Instead of walking your feet back, walk your hands forwards into a press-up position. Keeping your knees straight, walk your feet towards your hands until you feel a stretch in your hamstrings. Walk your hands forwards to begin the next repetition. You will be moving around the rooms during this exercise, so give yourself plenty of space.

DROP LUNGE

PROCEDURE:

Reach your left foot 60 centimetres (2 feet) behind your right foot. Square your hips back to the starting position, and sit back and down into a squat. Stand and step laterally with your right foot, then repeat the stretch on the same side. Continue until you've completed your reps on that side, then reverse directions and repeat.

COACHING KEY:

Keep your chest up and sit your hips back. Maintain your weight on the heel of your front leg. You will be moving around the room during this exercise, so give yourself plenty of space.

YOU SHOULD FEEL:

A stretch in the outsides of both hips.

WWW.COREPERFORMANCE.COM

PILLAR BRIDGE FRONT (KNEELING)

PROCEDURE:

Lying on your stomach with your forearms on the ground under your chest, push off your elbows, supporting your weight on your forearms and knees. Hold a static position for the prescribed length of time. Push your neck and sternum as far up and away from your forearms as possible.

COACHING KEY:

Keep your stomach tight.

YOU SHOULD FEEL IT:

In your shoulders and trunk.

PILLAR BRIDGE FRONT

PROCEDURE:

Same procedure as for Level 1, but instead of finishing with your knees on the floor, end in a prone press-up position, with just your forearms and toes resting on the floor. Push your chest as far away from the ground as possible. Hold your position for the prescribed amount of time.

COACHING KEY:

Keep your tummy tight and your head in line with your spine. There should be a straight line between your ear and your ankle, with no sagging or bending.

PILLAR BRIDGE FRONT (WIDE FEET)

PROCEDURE:

Once in the Pillar Bridge Front position, lift one arm, hold for 2 seconds. Switch arms. Widen your feet, if necessary, to reduce difficulty.

PILLAR BRIDGE FRONT (NARROW FEET)

PROCEDURE:

Same exercise as in Level 3. This time, narrow your feet to add to the degree of difficulty.

PREHAB

WWW.COREPERFORMANCE.COM

PILLAR BRIDGE LATERAL (KNEELING)

PROCEDURE:

Lie on your side with your forearm on the ground and your elbow under your shoulder, with your knees bent to 90 degrees. Push your forearm away from your body, lifting your hips into the air and supporting your weight on your forearm and knees. Hold a static position for the prescribed amount of time. Complete the reps on one side, then switch to the other side.

COACHING KEY:

Keep your body in a straight line and keep your stomach tight. If this is too difficult, do individual repetitions – 1 repetition per 2 seconds.

YOU SHOULD FEEL IT:

In your shoulders and trunk.

PREHAB

PILLAR BRIDGE LATERAL

PROCEDURE:

Lie on your side with your forearm on the ground under your shoulder, your feet split with the top leg forwards. With your body in a straight line and your elbow under your shoulder, push your hip off the ground, creating a straight line from ankle to shoulder and keeping your head in line with your spine. Hold your position for the pre-scribed amount of time.

PILLAR BRIDGE LATERAL (STACKED FEET)

PROCEDURE:

Instead of splitting your feet, stack them together.

PILLAR BRIDGE LATERAL (JUMPING JACK)

PROCEDURE:

From the bridge position, lift your top leg into the air as if you were doing a lateral jumping jack.

GLUTE BRIDGE (MINI BAND)

PROCEDURE:

Place a mini band just above your knees. Lying face up on the ground with your arms to your sides, your knees bent and your heels on the ground, lift your hips off the ground until your knees, hips and shoulders are in a straight line. Hold for the prescribed time. If this is too difficult, divide the time into 2- to 3-second intervals, then return to the starting position and repeat until you've completed all of your prescribed time.

COACHING KEY:

Fire (squeeze) your glutes.

YOU SHOULD FEEL IT:

In your glutes, and to a lesser degree in your hamstrings and lower back.

PREHAB

GLUTE BRIDGE (PADDED)

PROCEDURE:

Squeeze a rolled-up towel, a doubled-over Thera-Band pad or even a ball between your knees. Lift your hips into the air and then return to the starting position. Repeat for the prescribed number of reps.

GLUTE BRIDGE (MARCHING)

PROCEDURE:

Try 'marching' with one leg at a time.

GLUTE BRIDGE (KNEE BENT)

PROCEDURE:

Try to hold the Glute Bridge with one leg held to your chest and your weight supported on the other leg. Switch legs and repeat.

MINI BAND STANDING

PROCEDURE:

Stand with your feet just outside your hips and a mini band above your knees. Move into a partial squat. Keeping your left leg stationary, rotate your right knee in and out for the pre-scribed number of reps. Then switch legs and repeat on the other side.

COACHING KEY:

Keep both feet flat on the ground and your pelvis stable. Don't let the knee of your stationary leg drop inwards.

YOU SHOULD FEEL IT:

In your glutes.

LEVEL
2

MINI BAND WALKING

PROCEDURE:

Move to the right, pushing out with your left leg to create resistance while stepping laterally with your right leg. Bring your right foot back to the starting position and continue until you've completed your reps on that side. Be sure to keep your knees pushed apart throughout the movement. Repeat while moving to the left.

MINI BAND WALKING (ADD RESISTANCE)

PROCEDURE:

Increase the resistance by using a band with greater tension.

PREHAB

FLOOR *Y*S AND *T*S

PROCEDURE:

Lying face down on the floor with your arms raised slightly above shoulder height, create a *Y*, with your torso and arms, with your thumbs pointing up. Glide your shoulder blades towards your spine and lift your arms off the ground. Return to the starting position and repeat to complete your reps. For the *T*, pull your shoulder blades in towards your spine and extend your arms out to the sides so that they create a *T* with your torso.

COACHING KEY:

Keep your stomach tight and your thumbs up. Move from the scapulae (the shoulder blades), not from your arms, extending your shoulders and hands throughout the movement.

YOU SHOULD FEEL IT:

In your shoulders and upper back.

PHYSIOBALL *Y*S AND *T*S (ARMS BENT)

PROCEDURE:

Perform the same exercises with bent elbows on a physioball, lying face down over the top of the ball so that your back is flat and your chest is held up off the ball.

PHYSIOBALL *Y*S AND *T*S (ARMS EXTENDED)

PROCEDURE:

Perform the same exercise as for Level 2, but with your arms fully extended instead of bent.

PHYSIOBALL *Y*S AND *T*S (WITH WEIGHT)

PROCEDURE:

Add a light weight – 500 grams to 1.5 kilograms (1 to 3 lbs).

PREHAB

SUMO SQUAT to HAMSTRING STRETCH

PROCEDURE:

Standing with your feet shoulder width apart, bend at the waist and grab your toes. Drop your hips to the ground, lift your chest up and then pull your hips forwards until your torso is vertical. Maintaining a flat back, push your hips up and back until you feel a stretch in your hamstrings. Drop your hips back to the ground and repeat until you've completed all your reps.

COACHING KEY:

Keep your chest up, your back flat and your heels on the floor. Keep your elbows inside your knees. For an easier move, place a 1- to 5-centimetre ($\frac{1}{4}$- to 2-inch) block under your heels. As your mobility and stability improve, perform the movement with a smaller and smaller heel lift.

YOU SHOULD FEEL:

A stretch in your hamstrings, groin, lower back and quads.

PHYSIOBALL PLATE CRUNCH

PROCEDURE:

Holding a weight plate, lie on top of the ball and arch your torso backwards. Try to touch your shoulder blades, back and glutes to the ball so that your abdominals are completely stretched. Hold the weight plate behind your head. Roll your hips and chest up at the same time while pulling your belly button in. Crunch from the top of your torso and then lower your hips and chest to the starting position.

COACHING KEY:

Arch your torso completely.

YOU SHOULD FEEL:

A stretch in your abs and core.

PRESS-UP (KNEELING), OR **PRESS-UP**

PROCEDURE:

Assume a press-up position with your hands and knees on the ground. Lower your body to the ground, then reverse the movement without touching the ground. Keep your body in a straight line. If you don't need to kneel, assume the normal press-up position.

COACHING KEY:

Push your sternum as far away from your hands as possible at the end of the movement.

YOU SHOULD FEEL IT:

In your chest, arms and torso.

PRESS-UP (WITH PHYSIOBALL)

PROCEDURE:

Assume a press-up position, but with your hands on a physioball and your feet on the floor. With your belly button drawn in, lower yourself to the point where your chest just grazes the ball. Control the ball as you push back up, holding your belly button in and pushing your sternum as far away from the ball as possible. Your shoulder blades should be pushed away from each other in a 'plus' position (as far forwards as possible) at the top of the movement. Keep your fingers pointed down the sides of the ball.

STRENGTH

GLUTE BRIDGE (WITH PHYSIOBALL)

PROCEDURE:

Lie face up on the ground with your tummy tight and your feet on the ball (or on a bench or a couch). Your legs should be straight, your toes pulled up towards your shins and your shoulder blades pulled back and down. Contract your glutes to raise your hips until you create a straight line between your ankle and shoulders, so that only your head, shoulders and arms are touching the floor. Hold for 2 to 3 seconds and repeat until you've completed the prescribed number of reps.

COACHING KEY:

Initiate the movement by firing your glutes, and keep them contracted at the top of the movement. If it is too difficult to balance, spread your arms out to the side. Or, to make it more difficult, cross your arms on your chest.

YOU SHOULD FEEL IT:

In your glutes, hamstrings and in your lower back.

GLUTE BRIDGE (WITH PHYSIOBALL LEG CURL)

PROCEDURE:

Contract your glutes to raise your hips, then pull your heels towards your body. Do not let your hips drop as the ball comes towards you. Extend your legs, then repeat the leg curl for the prescribed number of reps without letting your hips touch the ground.

STRENGTH

FLOOR CRUNCH

PROCEDURE:

Lie face up with your knees bent, with a small pad or towel under your lower back to help stretch your abs, and your hands behind your head supporting your neck. Lift your chest until your shoulder blades are off the ground, and at the same time rotate your pelvis towards your belly button. Slowly return to the starting position. Repeat until you've completed your reps.

COACHING KEY:

Do not pull on your head with your hands. Feel each segment of your spine flexing as you crunch and as you stretch over the pad.

YOU SHOULD FEEL IT:

In your abdominals.

PHYSIOBALL CRUNCH

PROCEDURE:

Lie face up with your body arched over the ball and your hands interlocked, supporting your head. Drape your body over the ball – you should feel a mild stretch in your abs. Curl your trunk and pelvis together while keeping your belly button pulled in. Return to the starting position and repeat until you've completed all your reps.

STRENGTH

SQUAT (BODY WEIGHT, WITH MINI BAND)

PROCEDURE:

Stand with your arms at your sides, your feet shoulder width apart and pointing straight ahead, and a mini band around and above your knees. Maintain perfect posture and initiate movement with your hips. As you reach your arms far forwards, squat your hips back and down until your thighs are parallel to the floor. Return to a standing position by pushing through your hips. Keep your knees out. Repeat until you've completed all your reps.

COACHING KEY:

Keep your knees behind your toes during the movement. Also, keep your knees pushing out against the band so that they do not collapse to the inside during the movement. If you extend your arms in front of you, you can sit back more comfortably. Keep your chest up and your back flat.

YOU SHOULD FEEL IT:

In your glutes, hamstrings and quads.

SQUAT (SINGLE LEG WITH WEIGHTS)

PROCEDURE:

Stand on one foot in front of a bench or chair, holding 1- to 2-kilogram (2½- to 5-lb) weights in each hand. Initiate movement with your hips, squatting back and down on one leg as you reach forwards until your glutes touch the bench. Return to a standing position using only the leg you are balancing on. Repeat for the prescribed number of repetitions, then switch legs. Do not let your knee collapse to the inside.

SPLIT SQUAT

PROCEDURE:

Hold dumbbells at arm's length at your sides. Place one foot on a box or bench and step out with the other foot into a lunge. Lower your hips towards the floor by squatting back and down. Without letting your back knee touch the ground, return to the starting position by driving your weight back up with your front leg. Do all the reps with that leg forwards, then switch legs and repeat with the other leg forwards.

COACHING KEY:

Don't let your front knee slide forwards over your toes; if it does, start the movement over again with your front foot further forwards.

YOU SHOULD FEEL IT:

In your hips and the fronts of your legs.

SPLIT DUMBBELL CURL

PROCEDURE:

In a standing position, hold dumbbells at your side and place one leg on a stable object at about mid-thigh height. Shift your weight forwards onto your front leg, taking your back leg into a stretch. Now, keeping your elbows still, lift the dumbbells to your shoulders as you rotate your palms to the ceiling. Return to the starting position and repeat until you've completed all your reps. Switch legs mid-way through the set.

COACHING KEY:

Keep your stomach and the glute muscles of your rear leg tight throughout the movement. Do not allow your back to move. Do not rock forwards or backwards, and don't move your elbows.

YOU SHOULD FEEL IT:

In your biceps, glutes and hip flexors.

SPLIT DUMBBELL CURL TO PRESS

PROCEDURE:

After performing a biceps curl, press the weight over your head, finishing with your palms facing forwards. Switch legs midway through the set.

WWW.COREPERFORMANCE.COM

ALTERNATING SPLIT DUMBBELL CURL TO PRESS

PROCEDURE:

Stand holding dumbbells at your sides with your front foot resting on a bench or sturdy step at about mid-thigh height. Push your body weight slightly forwards, with your back glute tight. Perform a biceps curl so that the dumbbells are at your chest. Press your right hand over your head as you lower the left hand back to your side. As you lower your right hand, repeat the motion with your left arm so that the dumbbells pass at your torso. Repeat for the prescribed number of repetitions, switching the foot on the bench halfway through the set. Contract the glute of your back leg to stabilize yourself. Switch legs midway through the set.

COACHING KEY:

Maintain perfect posture, with your belly button pulled in and your shoulder blades pulled back and down. Do not let your back arch when the weight is pressed overhead.

YOU SHOULD FEEL IT:

In your biceps and shoulders and throughout your pillar.

STANDING LIFT

PROCEDURE:

Squat, rotating from right to left while holding a weight plate. Then rotate right, rising back to an upright position, before continuing to rotate and raising the weight plate over your head.

COACHING KEY:

Keep your chest up and your back flat. This exercise combines the familiar movements of squatting, rotating, the upright row and the incline press. Lower your body and the weight in the same pattern as you lifted.

YOU SHOULD FEEL IT:

In your hips, torso rotators, upper back, chest and shoulders.

STANDING LIFT (ONE LEG)

PROCEDURE:

Stand holding a weight plate or dumbbell in a low position, or holding a rope handle attached to a low pulley cable. Your foot should be perpendicular to the cable if you are using one, your hips should be flexed and your abdominals should be drawn in. Balance on your inside foot, turn your shoulders and hip towards the leg that's supporting your weight, and keep your chest up and your stomach tight. Squat down so that the weight is outside this leg, then fire from your glutes and torso. Pull the weight or handles towards your chest while extending your supporting leg. Turn your trunk away from your supporting leg as your hands push up and away. Return to the starting position and repeat to complete your reps, then switch legs.

COACHING KEY:

Keep your chest up and your back flat. Your torso will rotate from start to finish. This exercise combines the familiar movements of balance squatting, rotating, the upright row and the incline press. Lower in the same pattern as you lifted.

YOU SHOULD FEEL IT:

In your hips, torso rotators, upper back, chest and shoulders.

STRENGTH

ALTERNATING DUMBBELL BENCH PRESS

PROCEDURE:

Lie face up on a bench, holding dumbbells at the outside edges of your shoulders, your palms facing your thighs. Lift the dumbbells straight up over your chest. Keeping one arm straight, lower the other dumbbell, touch the outside of your shoulder, then push it back up. Switch arms and continue to alternate arms for the prescribed number of repetitions.

COACHING KEY:

Keep your non-working arm straight. Keep your feet on the floor and your hips and shoulders on the bench at all times. Pull your stomach in to stabilize your core.

YOU SHOULD FEEL IT:

In your chest, shoulders and triceps.

ROMANIAN DEADLIFT (TWO ARMS, ONE LEG)

PROCEDURE:

Stand on one foot while holding a dumbbell in each hand, using an overhand grip. 'Hinge' over at the waist, lowering the dumbbells as your non-supporting leg lifts behind you. Return to the standing position by contracting your hamstrings and glutes. Repeat for the prescribed number of repetitions, then switch legs.

COACHING KEY:

Do not let your back arch. Your torso and leg should move as one unit. Fire the glute of your extended leg to keep it straight. Keep your shoulder blades back and down throughout the movement, and keep the dumbbells close to your shin.

YOU SHOULD FEEL IT:

In your glutes, hamstrings and back.

STRENGTH

ONE-ARM, ONE-LEG DUMBBELL ROW

PROCEDURE:

Stand on your right leg, bent over at the waist, holding a dumbbell with your right hand and holding on to a stable, waist-high surface with your left hand. Lift your left leg to form a *T* with your body. Slide your right shoulder blade towards your spine and then lift the dumbbell to your body by driving your elbow to the ceiling. Return to the starting position and repeat for the prescribed number of repetitions. Then switch sides.

COACHING KEY:

Move with your shoulder, not your arm, to initiate the row. Keep your back level – your shoulders should stay parallel to the floor – and fire the glute of your extended leg to keep it parallel to the floor. Extend the leg opposite the hand doing the lifting.

YOU SHOULD FEEL IT:

In your back, lats and shoulders.

MINDSET

NUTRITION

MOVEMENT

RECOVERY

PART 4

CORE RECOVERY

AND

INTEGRATION

CHAPTER 11

REGENERATION

W hether it's working out or simply working at the office or at home, it's impossible to go all-out, all the time. You need some time to recover, a process I call regeneration.

Regeneration is a lifestyle philosophy, a recognition that you need to plan ways to recover – mentally and physically – in all areas of your life. You actually experience the benefit of your hard work on the days that you rest and repair your body.

There's a big difference between rest – doing nothing at all – and 'active rest'. In this programme, you work hard on Mondays, Wednesdays and Fridays, and devote Tuesdays and Thursdays to cardio work. If that's all that your schedule permits, fine – this programme was designed for the working person. It no doubt will take some effort to carve out time to work out on weekdays, and more likely than not, you won't have the time or inclination to exercise on the weekends.

I can appreciate that, and I applaud you for your efforts. But as you become more proficient with this programme, you might be looking for more. You could take some combination of Tuesday, Thursday, Saturday and Sunday and take a break from serious training but still do things that benefit your body,

WORK + REST = SUCCESS

Do you actively work recovery into your daily schedule? Into your yearly schedule?

Do you actively work recovery into your weekly exercise plan?

Do you understand the effective methods to recover, and do you allow your body to constantly regenerate to meet the demands of life?

such as playing golf, tennis or football. You're not training per se, but you're still getting the benefit of physical activity. Not only that, you're having fun too.

Regeneration is crucial for the body to experience the gains it made by working out. It's why we're not going to train superhard every day of the week, and it's why we'll take 48-hour breaks before revisiting elements of the Core Workout.

First, ask yourself the three questions above in 'Work + Rest = Success'.

'Regen' is not just a physical philosophy. The time spent at rest is when we enjoy the fruits of our labour. Not only that, but we also recharge our batteries and come back invigorated and stronger, ready to perform at even higher levels.

If you're working hard all the time, you're never truly recovered. You might be working hard, but you're not working smart. On the contrary – you're so mentally and physically fatigued that you're not nearly as productive as you think you are.

Remember, this programme will only be moderately successful if you have a limiting lifestyle, and for many people that limitation comes in the form of a lack of sleep. Sleep is a vital component of regeneration.

I see this even with elite athletes, especially younger ones. They have boundless energy and live nocturnal lifestyles, partying into the wee hours and getting little sleep. But even if they don't drink excessively, a couple of beers or cocktails inhibit sleep and contribute to weight gain.

While on the topic of alcohol, remember that earlier we discussed the health benefits of *moderate* consumption of red wine. But remember also that it's difficult to reap the full rewards of this programme if recreational drinking is a key part of your current lifestyle. (It goes without saying that smoking is counterproductive to healthy living.)

Sleep, though, is the most underrated aspect of a healthy lifestyle. Recent studies suggest that the less sleep you get, the more likely you are to be obese. Sleep deprivation

'The ability to do the things I've always wanted to do'

NAME: SOREN ORLEY

AGE: 49

OCCUPATION: CHARTERED ACCOUNTANT

Soren Orley had always maintained an active lifestyle. A keen climber who spends many weekends working for his local mountain rescue group, he prided himself on his fitness, even though he had put on some extra weight in his forties.

In June 2004, for his 48th birthday, his wife gave him a bicycle. He began riding frequently, only to put on a mysterious 5.4 kilograms (12 pounds) in less than a week. Though he felt queasy and short of breath, he chalked it up to being allergic to cats.

When he went to see his doctor, he was diagnosed him with an enlarged heart and pulmonary hypertension, probably a congenital defect. His body was retaining fluid. Two weeks later, Orley underwent surgery to repair an aortic valve.

While undergoing the hospital's rehabilitation programme and waiting 7 weeks for clearance to begin strenuous physical activity, Orley read *Core Performance*. He figured it was the right programme for him, especially after watching more advanced rehabilitation patients go through 'what seemed like a pretty wimpy programme.'

The medical staff gave him clearance, and within 3 months, his weight dropped to 87 kilograms (192 pounds), down from a high of 110 kilograms (241 pounds) before the surgery. He bought trousers with an 85-centimetre (34-inch) waist – 10 centimetres (4 inches) narrower than before. But the more telling results came in his improved flexibility and balance, especially while climbing.

'Before, if we were carrying an injured person on a stretcher in difficult conditions, I might have needed to take a break,' says Orley, a chartered accountant, 'Now I'm able to keep going. It's the little things that you notice most about the programme.'

Orley is back on duty with the rescue group, which sometimes requires hiking long distances with a 24-kilogram (65-pound) pack strapped to his back. 'When you're hanging off the side of a mountain in a storm, trying to keep people alive, you need all of the strength, balance and flexibility you can muster.'

Orley's biggest reward came in the summer of 2005, when one of his daughters graduated from university and he joined her on a cycling and climbing tour. In the course of a week, they cycled 320 kilometres (200 miles) and climbed a 1,220-m (4,000-foot) mountain.

Not bad at all for a guy who had major open-heart surgery less than a year ago.

'It's not just about how much weight you can lift or how many pounds you lose', Orley says of the Core Performance Programme. 'Those things are meaningful, but more important, this programme has given me the ability to do the things I've always wanted to do.'

decreases levels of a hormone called leptin that makes you feel full, and it increases levels of a hunger hormone called ghrelin. It's yet another vicious cycle: less sleep makes you fat, and being fat impedes your sleep. It is estimated that 63 per cent of adults don't get the recommended 8 hours of sleep a night. Sleep deprivation and sleep disorders cost millions annually in lost productivity, sick leave and medical expenses.

For all the talk of improving diet and exercise, we tend to ignore this obvious lifestyle component. Throughout this programme, I want you to make the best use of your time and get the most benefit, whether it's working out, eating or even sleeping. You probably know you should get 8 hours of sleep a night. But you might not know that it's possible to improve the quality of your sleep by thinking in terms of 90-minute cycles.

The longer you're asleep, the longer you experience rapid-eye-movement (REM) sleep, a period marked by increased brain activity and muscle relaxation. Sleep cycles last approximately 90 minutes, and at the end of each cycle, you start to come out of sleep as your body senses whether or not it can go into another sleep cycle.

If you're awakened in the middle of a sleep cycle by an alarm clock, a dream or a loud noise, you tend to be disoriented for a short while and end up feeling sluggish for much of the day. But if you can manage to wake up at the top of a 90-minute cycle, perhaps with the use of an alarm clock or because of daylight, you'll feel more alert and invigorated.

Sleeping 6 hours might feel more restful than 7 hours if you get up at the top of a sleep cycle. Ideally, you should aim for 7½ to 8 hours, but since many people struggle to get 6 hours of sleep, let's recognize that 6 hours of sleep can be a good thing – provided it's 6 hours of quality sleep, not sleep affected by alcohol – or by sugary foods eaten not long before bedtime.

On the following pages, we've provided some effective regeneration-oriented exercises to use in combination with the rest of the Core Workout routines. By using two simple pieces of equipment – a foam roll and a stretch rope – you can achieve some tremendous results. Using the foam roll is like having a massage. It uses deep compression to help roll out the muscle spasms that develop over time. The rope routine is especially helpful with flexibility. You need not think of the foam roll and rope routine as additional work; just use them while watching TV or at the end of the day, before going to bed.

Begin a pattern of rest and regeneration to balance all the challenging aspects of your life on a daily, weekly and yearly basis, and you'll be amazed at how high the quality of your life becomes.

Chapter 11 Summary: The process of regeneration requires the recognition that you need to plan ways to recover in all areas of your life – not just the physical. That way, you'll experience the benefit of the work you do as part of the Core Workout on the days you rest. (Remember: Work + Rest = Success.) The time spent at rest is when we clear our minds and enjoy the fruits of our labour, when we realize the gains produced by all of our hard work. Not only that, we also recharge our batteries and come back invigorated and stronger, ready to perform at even higher levels. Sleep is a vital component of regeneration. And proper nutrition is vital to the process, as it helps the body to regenerate effectively.

SELF-MASSAGE ROUTINE

FOAM ROLL QUADRICEPS/HIP FLEXOR

Lie face down on the floor with a foam roll under the front of your thighs. Roll over the quads from your hip to just above your knee. For added benefit, cross one leg over the other, placing all your body weight on the front of one thigh. The more uncomfortable it feels, the more that muscle needs to be massaged. Hold your position on sore spots for an extended time to release the soreness. Roll slightly on the outside and inside of the thighs as well as down the front of the thighs.

FOAM ROLL HAMSTRING

Sit on the floor and place a foam roll under the back of one thigh with your other leg crossed. Roll over the foam, moving it up and down the length of the back of your thigh. If it is too sensitive, uncross your legs and roll both hamstrings at once. The more uncomfortable it is, the more that muscle needs to be massaged. Hold your position on sore spots for an extended time to release the soreness, as if you were getting a massage.

FOAM ROLL I.T. BAND

Lie on your side with a foam roll under the outside of your thigh. Roll over the foam from your hip to just above your knee. The more uncomfortable it is, the more that muscle needs to be massaged. Hold your position on sore spots for an extended time to release the soreness, as if you were getting a massage.

FOAM ROLL LOWER BACK

Lie face up with a foam roll under your mid-back. Cross your arms over your chest. Roll from the middle of your back down to the base of your spine and repeat. The more uncomfortable it is, the more that muscle needs to be massaged. Hold your position on sore spots for an extended time to release the soreness, as if you were getting a massage.

FOAM ROLL UPPER BACK

Lie face up with a foam roll under your upper back. Hold your hands behind your head with your elbows pointed to the sky. Roll from your shoulders down to the middle of your back and repeat. The more uncomfortable it is, the more that muscle needs to be massaged. Hold your position on sore spots for an extended time to release the soreness, as if you were getting a massage.

FOAM ROLL LATS

Lie on your side with a foam roll under your armpit. Roll from the side of your lower back up to your armpit. The more uncomfortable it is, the more that muscle needs to be massaged. Hold your position on sore spots for an extended time to release the soreness, as if you were getting a massage.

FLEXIBILITY ROUTINE

ARCH ROLL (TENNIS BALL)

Standing with your shoes off, place one foot on a tennis ball. Roll the arch of your foot back and forth over the tennis ball. The more uncomfortable it is, the more that muscle needs to be massaged. Hold your position on sore spots for an extended time to release the soreness. Roll through different angles to cover the entire arch completely, as if you were getting a deep massage.

ROPE STRETCH – STRAIGHT LEG HAMSTRING

Lie on your back with your left leg straight and a rope wrapped around your foot. Actively lift your left leg as far as possible, then give it gentle assistance with the rope until a stretch is felt. Hold for 2 seconds and then relax. Repeat. Keep the opposite leg on the floor by pushing your heel as far away from your head as possible, contracting the glute. You should feel a stretch in the hamstring of your raised leg and a stretch in the hip flexor of your bottom leg.

ROPE STRETCH – BENT-KNEE HAMSTRING

Lie on your back with your left knee pulled to your chest and a rope wrapped around your foot. Actively straighten your left knee as much as possible without letting it move away from your chest, pulling the rope above your head. It is okay if the knee is not able to straighten fully. Give it gentle assistance with the rope until a stretch is felt, hold for 2 seconds, and then relax. Repeat for the prescribed number of repetitions.

QUAD/HIP FLEXOR STRETCH (KNEELING, BACK FOOT UP)

Place your back knee on a soft mat or pad with your back foot elevated on a chair or a physio-ball. While keeping a slight forward lean of the torso, tighten the core and the glute of the leg with the knee on the ground. Maintaining this posture, shift your entire body slightly forwards. Exhale and hold the stretch for 2 seconds. Relax and repeat. Avoid excessive arching in your back. You should feel a stretch in the front of your hip and your upper thigh.

90/90 STRETCH

Lie face up on the floor with your arms out to the side, your left knee bent to 90 degrees and your right leg crossed over the left. Roll over onto your left side, pinning a pad between your right knee and the ground. While maintaining pressure on the pad and keeping your hips still, rotate your chest and right arm back to the right, trying to put your back on the ground. Hold for 2 seconds and then return to the starting position. Repeat, and then switch sides.

GLUTE STRETCH (SUPINE)

Lying face up on the ground, actively lift one knee to your chest and then give it gentle assistance by grabbing the knee and pulling it closer to your chest. Exhale and hold the stretch for 2 seconds, then return to the starting position. Repeat, and then switch legs. Keep your non-stretching leg flat on the floor by pushing the bottom of your heel away from your head. You should feel a stretch in your glutes, hamstrings and hip flexors.

QUALITY OF TIME

f you've ever watched an hourglass, you've witnessed an optical illusion. At first, the sand seems to pass through the narrow opening slowly. But the more sand passes through, the faster it seems to progress.

The same is true with time. The older we get, the more quickly time appears to pass. We know that this is not *literally* true, but the fast-pace of adult life means that time seems to fly by more quickly than what we remember as children, when the last hour of the school day or the final weeks before the winter holidays seemed to go on forever.

Time is a limiting factor for everyone and can be the biggest obstacle to leading a healthy lifestyle. After all, everyone wants to exercise, but they can't find the time. Everyone wants to eat healthier meals, but they only have time to grab something quick. Everyone wants to get more sleep and rely less on caffeine, but who has the time?

Now that we've addressed these challenges, we need to look at time from a broader perspective. We need a framework to execute these new strategies. Everything we do within our Core Essentials sphere will only work if it's an integrated lifestyle.

Most of us purchase day planners and desk calendars in December, mapping out all of the important events for the following year. These days, it's possible to do it all electronically.

In theory, this exercise is supposed to provide structure and organization to our lives, and to some degree it does. But it also causes us to look short-term, at the upcoming day or week, and be reactive, like a goalie.

Instead, why don't we map out the year on one sheet of paper? (See the planning calendars provided on pages 198 and 199.) You can still use your daily or weekly planners, but it will be easier to concentrate on the most important things and find chunks of time where you can make a difference.

This calendar shows Monday through to Sunday at a glance. This will help you be more proactive. Take a highlighter and block out the week between Christmas and New Year and any weeklong holidays in the school calendar if you have children or are a student yourself.

When you do this, it not only makes things seem more manageable, but it enables you to see smaller 6-week and 8-week windows where you can set up process-oriented goals. For instance, for the first 6-week block, we already have set realistic goals of working out three times a week, along with purging your cupboards of unhealthy foods and stocking them with better choices.

Break this 6-week block into chunks, adapting it to your lifestyle. Otherwise, it might seem overwhelming. You might think, 'I've got a trip coming up in March, and then the children are on holidays in April, and we're travelling at Easter this year. There's just no way'.

If you break up the time, your plan doesn't seem so impossible. It also speaks to the key component of recovery. You can't work out diligently or go to the office 7 days a week, every week. Your body and soul would not allow it. You have to know that there's some built-in reward in the form of weekends and holiday. That time allows you to recharge and come back even stronger.

Think of how hard you work before a holiday. You scramble to make sure everything is done at the office and that someone covers for you in the event that something comes up in your absence. At home, you put the house in order, arrange for pet care and stop the post and newspapers. You move at a furious pace because of that dangling carrot of a holiday.

The same is true with this programme. If you know there's a break in the workout routine or a break in your schedule, in the form of holiday, it will inspire you to work that much more efficiently during your workouts.

No matter how we structure our lives, we have to work hard. Vince Lombardi, a legendary American football coach, once famously remarked that 'the only place success comes before work is in the dictionary'. This is as true of physical fitness as it is of other successes.

No matter how proactive we are in terms of scheduling and structuring our lives, there will be things we can't control. There's a part of every day where you just have to stand up to the demands of life, even if that means

'I'm outdriving the boys!'

NAME: JANET OJA

AGE: 44

OCCUPATION: MEDICAL EQUIPMENT TECHNICIAN

Janet Oja always considered herself a pretty good athlete. The Core programme alleviated some recurring shoulder problems, but the biggest benefit she received from the programme was finding the confidence to try sports that require not only core strength but also mental toughness.

These days, she enjoys 'canyoneering', exploring canyons near her home through a combination of hiking, swimming, abseiling and rock climbing.

'I had always wanted to try rock climbing, but, like a lot of women, I didn't think that I had the upper body strength,' she says. 'Now I know that anyone can generate this tremendous core strength, no matter what they begin with.'

Not long after starting the programme, she began to outpace her husband on bicycle rides. She noticed while hiking that her balance was significantly better. Climbing hills was much easier. The most telling sign came when she started outdriving her male counterparts on the golf course.

'I always thought I was centred and balanced on the golf course, but now I'm not falling off the back of my shoes,' says Oja, who works as a medical equipment technician. 'I feel the difference constantly, whether I'm picking up a bag of shopping or if I slip while hiking. Now, I automatically catch myself and don't miss a beat.

'It's like rediscovering sport all over again. Every time I participate in a sport, whether I've done it before or not, I always anticipate how the Core programme has enhanced how well I "play". I am never disappointed.'

Oja, who does her core training in a spare bedroom at home, has been so successful that she has introduced the programme to her two sons, who play football and baseball. Having completed marathons and triathlons in the past, she's hardly lacking in competitive drive, but she says her core training has given her the confidence to attempt anything physical.

'Even in my forties, I can still pick up new things, which is amazing,' she says. 'This programme has allowed me to dream bigger when it comes to sports.'

playing goalie. I run several successful businesses, with employees and clients that require attention, and some days I find that I'm busy just putting out fires.

The key is to improve our efficiency – our quality of time – and work smarter. A friend of mine once gave me a terrific compliment, saying he was continually amazed by my ability to show a greater capacity for work. At first, I was taken aback. I make it a priority to spend time with family and friends and on things I enjoy. I don't think of myself as a workaholic.

But what my friend meant was that I find a way to get more done in the same period of time; I continually work more efficiently – and it starts with my health. No matter how busy I become, I know that I must get that daily exercise in and eat properly.

So, I schedule that time like any other appointment. In addition to my one-sheet, 365-day calendar, I keep a weekly calendar that includes a weekday workout at 6:15 a.m. I exercise for no more than 60 minutes, and usually just 30, but I'm able to make that workout progressively more efficient and thus more effective as time passes.

For many people, the only time to work out will be the first thing in the morning. That sets a good tone for the rest of the day and provides you with a powerful endorphin rush to tackle the tasks ahead. For stay-at-home parents, that's the worst time of day since there are children who need attention. Perhaps you can

schedule your workout around school or naptime. (If that's too unpredictable, a growing number of fitness chains provide the equivalent of 1- or 2-hour daycare right in the gym.)

No matter how busy you are, there is a window of opportunity. Start by looking at the broad, year-long picture. Set some manageable goals, and then find that one period of the day where you can make it happen, and schedule it. This is no different from what I do with professional athletes. We take their year-long daily schedules of practice and games, and work in training around it.

I know, I know; if you had an exciting, high-paying job contingent on being in top physical condition, you too would feel inspired to work out harder. But here's the funny little secret of my business: most athletes, because of the gruelling travel and rigid schedule of competition and practices, plus family, do not have much time for day-to-day conditioning. The reason they are world class is that they find the time in their day.

That's great for my business since they take advantage of 4- to 6-week visits to my facilities for some intense training. The rest of the year, we support them with programmes to maintain their bodies throughout the season.

When you look at your year-long calendar, you will find periods where it might be impossible to do much. The key is to have a programme in place where you can do *something* during those periods and then be focused the rest of the time.

The goal, of course, is to have goals, not to just play goalkeeper. How many times does New Year's Eve roll around and we wonder where the year went and what we have to show for it? It's like the person who has worked in the same position for 15 years. Has his career seen steady progression, or does he just have 1 year of experience repeated 15 times over?

We don't just want to maintain our lives; we want to constantly make them more efficient and productive so that we can enjoy more. It starts with our physical health. Our bodies are the vehicles for our success, and it's a lot eas-ier to stay motivated when you know that it's not just about you. As a centred self, it's about how you can help and elevate others.

Chapter 12 Summary: We want to make the most of our time by looking at the calendar in terms of manageable chunks of time. Whether finding time to work out or looking to fit in all of our work and personal commitments, we want to find windows of opportunity and set man-ageable goals that can be achieved. You'll find that within this structure you can accomplish almost anything.

2006 ANNUAL PLANNING CALENDAR

EVENT	MONDAY	TUESDAY	WEDNESDAY	THURSDAY	FRIDAY	SATURDAY	SUNDAY
JAN 2							
9							
16							
23							
30							
FEB 6							
13							
20							
27							
MAR 6							
13							
20							
27							
APR 3							
10							
17							
24							
MAY 1							
8							
15							
22							
29							
JUN 5							
12							
19							
26							
JUL 3							
10							
17							
24							
31							
AUG 7							
14							
21							
28							
SEP 4							
11							
18							
25							
OCT 2							
9							
16							
23							
30							
NOV 6							
13							
20							
27							
DEC 4							
11							
18							
25							

2007 ANNUAL PLANNING CALENDAR

EVENT	MONDAY	TUESDAY	WEDNESDAY	THURSDAY	FRIDAY	SATURDAY	SUNDAY
JAN 1							
8							
15							
22							
29							
FEB 5							
12							
19							
26							
MAR 5							
12							
19							
26							
APR 2							
9							
16							
23							
30							
MAY 7							
14							
21							
28							
JUN 4							
11							
18							
25							
JUL 2							
9							
16							
23							
30							
AUG 6							
13							
20							
27							
SEP 3							
10							
17							
24							
OCT 1							
8							
15							
22							
29							
NOV 5							
12							
19							
26							
DEC 3							
10							
17							
24							
31							

CHAPTER 13

KEEPING SCORE

n my previous book, *Core Performance,* we issued a challenge to readers to send us their feedback about the programme. The greatest reward of writing that book was that I got to hear from people who used the Core system to overcome pain, lose weight, increase their flexibility and install a plan of high-performance nutrition and exercise for long-term health and success.

You've heard from some of those people in this book. We brought others out to our Athletes' Performance training facility in Tempe, Arizona, for a special week of training so they could share with me first-hand how the Core programme has affected their lives.

Thousands of people have joined our online community at *www.coreperformance.com*. Each week, we answer their questions about the Core programme and provide them with the latest scientific information on nutrition, fitness and performance. I hope you'll join this growing community of people who have made the commitment to a lifetime of high performance health and well-being.

This is an ongoing process. You'll notice that we didn't put a time frame on this programme. There was no '12 Weeks to a Better You' slogan, no '6-Week Plan for Success' subtitle. We presented *Core Performance* as a 12-week plan because, well, that's what everyone in the world of fitness book publishing tends to do. We found that most people wanted more. They didn't wish to repeat the 12-week cycle or the latter stages; they were looking for more progression beyond the 12 weeks.

We assembled this programme with the goal of using as little equipment as possible. We wanted to eliminate excuses for not working out, while providing an efficient programme that will allow you to succeed regardless of your financial resources. By following this programme, you will achieve great results.

But perhaps you have a little more money to spend. And, if you do, there are some tools we provide that can help you train even more efficiently to thrive in the Game of Life.

Our Web site, *www.coreperformance.com*, is the home for the products and programmes we have developed and tested that will complement your Core training programme.

First, check out our online Core Store. We have assembled several tools, based on the book, that are great resources for the Core Performance Essentials programme, whether you prefer to work out at home or in a gym. The shop can ship equipment internationally, and can give you a good idea of what to look for in your local sports shop. One thing you won't find in your local shop is the Core Performance Essentials DVD series, in which I lead you through the various 30-minute workouts right in your living room.

Alternatively, you'll find in the Core Store a set of laminated cards featuring each level of the workouts with exercise pictures. These cards are a great tool to remind you of proper form as you work out at home or the gym.

Also in the Core Store, we have assembled several packages to create a Core Gym at home. I know that you are incredibly busy, and maybe a gym membership is just not feasible or maybe you have a membership but are never able to use it for lack of time. A simple Core home gym lets you build the Core programme around *your* life.

Maybe you're thinking, 'Sure, that would be great, but I don't have the time or space for elaborate equipment'. The beauty of this programme is that the equipment is compact and easy to use.

Our equipment partner, GoFit, has compiled several affordable packages of equipment that you can purchase with a single click in the Core Store. As I said before, our shop does ship internationally, but you should be able to find similar equipment in most sports shops.

Once you've checked out the Core Store, you will notice a whole world of Core Performance programmes available on the Web site. If you're new to the Core Performance community and just getting the hang of taking charge of your body and your life, I want you to focus on this book and mastering the programme. We tried to make this book all-encompassing, and if you just keep trying to pack more and more into your 30-minute workouts, this book might be all you ever need.

But if you're someone who wants to commit a little more time, or if you've caught the Core 'bug' and want to take your game to higher levels, check out the programmes available.

These programmes include the original *Core Performance* book and the supplemental CD-ROM, along with sport-specific DVD training systems for golf, football, tennis and other sports. Each of these DVDs contains a programme with more than 60 exercises designed in a programme to help you prepare to thrive in each of these sports. These are great products if you're a competitive or recreational athlete, and I have even recommended them with great success to professional athletes who cannot join us at our Athletes' Performance facilities.

I also recommend that you check out our powerful interactive platform, which can be accessed from *www.coreperformance.com*. We created this platform based on feedback from readers of the original *Core Performance* who were looking to progress beyond the basic 12-week programme. This interactive platform features Core Performance programmes for every level of fitness and every major sport. My staff and I assembled these programmes in a powerful database, all customized to your goals, interests and life's demands according to your answers to some simple questions.

The Web site a complete nutritional system that complements your customized training programme, providing you with recommendations on meal timing and food choices as part of your customized 'Perfect Day' routine. We have effective visual tools that let you monitor your progress. There are video clips of every exercise. And I try to provide you with daily tips and world-class content that reflect the constantly evolving research and development we do at Athletes' Performance every day.

In short, *www.coreperformance.com* is the next best thing to being here in person.

Ultimately, I want you to be members of the Core Performance online community for life, which is why we have made a full-year membership available for less than the monthly cost of a gym membership. This means that for very little money, you will have access to progressive programmes that are based upon your accomplishments and that can change with you as your goals and the demands on your time change.

Even better, because you already have made a commitment to joining the Core community, I am providing you with a free 3-week trial to try out the site. From *www.coreperformance.com*, simply click on 'Enter Your Access Code' and type in the following code: CPE20495. You'll then have 3 weeks to sample all of the programmes, check out all of the amazing tools on the site and decide whether you want to become a full member.

A further benefit of your interactive Web site membership – trial or actual – is that you can access our Video Library and view video clips of every exercise that is in the Core Performance Essentials programme. For those people who are visually oriented (and I'm one of them), these videos will help you to see the proper form for every exercise from two different angles. And as you know, it is important to do these exercises correctly to maximize the gain.

However you proceed from here, I hope you do so as a centred self. Operate with core values, with long-term health as your first priority, and you'll find that your body will become the vehicle for your success with family, at work and in everything you do. Remember to always think of yourself as an athlete competing in the Game of Life.

Don't look at this new lifestyle as a short-term solution. This is not a home renovation, something with a beginning and an end.

By making this investment in yourself, you improve not only your health but also your mental and spiritual outlook. You become a better spouse, a better parent, a better sibling. That means the lives of your loved ones improve as well.

Earlier in the book, you heard from Janet Oja, who said that this programme allowed her to 'dream bigger'. By mastering movements, eliminating pain, boosting energy and fuelling your body properly, you'll walk with a little more swagger and confidence. You'll glide through life, feeling as if you can master anything.

For Janet, that meant abseiling into canyons and climbing out by whatever means necessary. What's the equivalent of that in your life? What challenge would you like to meet?

I've had great success supporting people in the pursuit of their dreams. Some of them are prominent sporting figures, but many of them are people just like you who have reached spectacular goals. What I love most is being able to build my clients ability, to see them evolve and reach their goals.

We tend to keep score in the West with money. Whoever dies with the most toys wins, right? Wrong. The winner is the one who dies at a ripe old age, while still living an active life, having elevated others and built deep relationships along the way. I hope you'll keep score of your success within this programme – whatever your definition of success might be – not just by how much weight you've lost or how you look in the mirror, but by how the quality of your life has improved. You've heard from people in this book who have lost weight, but the most important thing was that they found more energy for their children and partners. And at Athletes' Performance, we've heard from others who have gained the confidence to pursue entrepreneurial endeavours, travel the world, or simply pursue a sport or physical activity that they never dared try before.

I'm excited about this book because I will get to hear from more people like you, and that inspires me. So many of you have become vocal advocates for this programme, and I can't tell you how much I appreciate that.

I'm blown away when I hear someone like Mike Dixey tell me that he's used this programme to overcome something like vertigo. Mike concluded his note with, 'Mark, you have truly made a significant impact on my life. Anytime you have a bad day or need a lift, please pull out this letter and read it'.

You bet I will, Mike.

I want to hear how this programme has transformed your life – and not just from a physical standpoint. Tell me how it has enabled you to meet challenges and fulfil your dreams. I want to hear about what you've overcome and the roadblocks you've navigated. Tell the entire Core community how taking a proactive approach to life has made a difference.

Please share your stories with us at *mark@coreperformance.com*. We'll pick the most inspirational submissions, the ones that touch us the most, and bring the authors of those remarks to Athletes' Performance to train in person with our staff, alongside some of the best athletes in the world.

Let's help each other stay motivated through the Web site, where I will track your progress based upon your goals. You will empower me through your achievements and your courage.

You can share with me personally how you've transformed your life to meet your goals.

We can't bring everyone out, unfortunately. I hope you join our online community and interact with the growing number of people dedicated to treating each day as an athletic event and properly preparing themselves for the competition that is the Game of Life.

Welcome to the Core.

Your coach,

Mark Verstegen

THE CORE WORKOUT AT A GLANCE

After my first book, *Core Performance,* we received a lot of suggestions from readers about how they would have preferred the exercises presented differently. Recognizing that people visualize and process information differently, we've laid out the exercises in three ways.

We've presented the Core Workout in a level-by-level format (pages 118 to 125) and in an exercise-by-exercise format (pages 126 to 178). With this appendix, I thought I'd combine the two and give you another at-a-glance view of the whole Core Workout. In all three versions, you'll see that while there are not that many exercises, the variations and progressions that you can make are virtually unlimited.

90/90 STRETCH

PROCEDURE: Lie on the ground on your left side in a foetal position, with your legs tucked up into your torso at a 90-degree angle and a pad or rolled-up towel between your knees. Keep both arms straight at a 90-degree angle to your torso. Now, keeping your knees together and on the ground and your hips still, rotate your chest and right arm back to the right, trying to put your back on the ground. Exhale and hold for 2 seconds, then return to the starting position. Finish your reps, then switch sides and repeat.

LEVEL 2

90/90 STRETCH (LEGS CROSSED)

PROCEDURE: Lie face up on the ground holding a pad or towel roll, your left knee bent to 90 degrees, and your right leg crossed over the left. Roll over onto your left side and pin the pad between your right knee and the ground. Maintaining pressure on the pad and keeping your hips still, rotate your chest and right arm back to the right, trying to put your back on the ground. Hold for 2 seconds, then return to the starting position. Repeat until you've completed your reps, then switch sides.

LEVEL 3

HIP CROSSOVER

PROCEDURE: Lie face up on the ground with your arms to your sides, your knees bent and your feet flat. Twist your bent legs to the left until they reach the floor, then twist them to the right. Continue for the prescribed number of repetitions.

LEVEL 4

HIP CROSSOVER (FEET UP)

PROCEDURE: Try this move with your hips and knees bent to 90 degrees and your feet held off the ground. Once you master that, perform this move with your legs straight.

WWW.COREPERFORMANCE.COM

LUNGE STRETCH

PROCEDURE: Take a half-step forwards with your left foot, placing your right hand on the floor for balance. Take your left elbow and reach down the inside of your forward leg until you feel a stretch. Then place your left hand on the floor and push your hips upwards as you straighten your front leg. Return to the starting position and repeat. **COACHING KEY:** Contract (squeeze) the glute muscle of your back leg. **YOU SHOULD FEEL:** A stretch through the groin, the hip flexor muscle of your back leg, and the glute muscle and hamstring of your front leg.

LUNGE STRETCH (BACKWARD)

PROCEDURE: With your feet together, step back with your right leg into a lunge. While reaching your right hand to the sky, bend your torso to the left. Straighten your torso and step forwards into the starting position. Alternate sides and repeat for the prescribed repetitions.

LUNGE STRETCH (MOVING)

PROCEDURE: Instead of returning to the starting position as in Level 2, walk forwards into the next position.

INVERTED HAMSTRING (IN PLACE)

PROCEDURE: Stand on one leg with perfect posture, holding on to a wall, chair or table for stability. Keep your shoulder blades back and down. Maintaining a straight line from ear to ankle, bend over at the waist, raising your opposite heel to the sky. When you feel a stretch, return to the standing position by contracting the muscles of your hamstring, glutes and back. Complete your reps on that side, then switch legs. **COACHING KEY:** Keep your back flat and your hips and shoulders parallel to the ground. Maintain a straight line from your ear through your hip, knee and ankle. Try to keep your balance without relying on your hand, and keep your opposite foot off the ground. **YOU SHOULD FEEL:** A stretch in your hamstrings.

INVERTED HAMSTRING (BACKWARD)

PROCEDURE: Complete on rep of the momemen (without a chair for support), then step back into the next step and repeat using the opposite leg, alternating legs until you've completed all your reps.

LATERAL LUNGE

PROCEDURE: Standing with your feet wider than shoulder width apart, shift your hips to the left and down by bending your left knee and keeping your right leg straight. Your feet should be straight ahead and flat on the ground. Push through your left hip, returning to the starting position. Alternate sides and repeat for the prescribed number of repetitions. **COACHING KEY:** Keep your knee on your 'working' side behind your toes. Keep your opposite leg straight, your back flat and your chest up. **YOU SHOULD FEEL:** A lengthening and strengthening of your glutes, groin, hamstrings and quads.

LEVEL 2

LATERAL LUNGE (STEP AND RETURN)

PROCEDURE: Step to the right with your right foot, keeping your toes forwards and your feet flat. Squat through your right hip while keeping your left leg straight. Squat as low as possible, holding this position for 2 seconds. Push back to the starting position and repeat to the opposite side.

LEVEL 2 & 4

LATERAL LUNGE (MOVING)

PROCEDURE: Instead of returning to the starting position, step into a squat position and then into the next lunge. Repeat for the prescribed number of repetitions and then switch sides. You will be stepping around the room during this exercise, so give yourself plenty of space.

LEVEL 2

HANDWALK (REVERSE)

PROCEDURE: Bend at the waist and walk your feet out into a press-up position. Now, keeping your knees straight, walk your hands towards your feet. When you feel a stretch, walk your feet back out to a press-up position. Repeat until you've completed your reps. **COACHING KEY:** Keep your knees straight and your stomach tight. Walk your hands out further beyond your head for increased difficulty. Use short 'ankle steps' to walk back up to your hands. That is, take baby steps using only your ankles – don't use your knees, hips or quads. **YOU SHOULD FEEL:** A stretch in your hamstrings, lower back, glutes and calves.

LEVEL 3&4

HANDWALK

PROCEDURE: Instead of walking your feet backwards, walk your hands forwards into a press-up position. Keeping your knees straight, walk your feet towards your hands until you feel a stretch in your hamstrings. Walk your hands forwards to begin the next repetition. You will be moving around the room during this exercise, so give yourself plenty of space.

DROP LUNGE

LEVEL 3 & 4

DROP LUNGE

PROCEDURE: Reach your left foot 60 centimetres (2 feet) behind your right foot. Square your hips back to the starting position, and sit back and down into a squat. Stand and step laterally with your right foot, then repeat the stretch on the same side. Continue until you've completed your reps on that side, then reverse directions. **COACHING KEY:** Keep your chest up and sit your hips back. Maintain your weight on the heel of your front leg. You will be moving around the room during this exercise, so give yourself plenty of space. **YOU SHOULD FEEL:** A stretch in the outsides of both hips.

PILLAR BRIDGE FRONT

PILLAR BRIDGE FRONT (KNEELING)

PROCEDURE: Lying on your stomach with your forearms on the ground under your chest, push off your elbows, supporting your weight on your forearms and knees. Hold a static position for the prescribed length of time. Push your neck and sternum as far up and away from your forearms as possible. **COACHING KEY:** Keep your stomach tight. **YOU SHOULD FEEL IT:** In your shoulders and trunk.

PILLAR BRIDGE FRONT

PROCEDURE: Same procedure as for Level 1, but instead of finishing with your knees on the floor, end in a prone press-up position, with just your forearms and toes resting on the floor. Push your chest as far away from the ground as possible. Hold your position for the prescribed amount of time. **COACHING KEY:** Keep your tummy tight and your head in line with your spine. There should be a straight line between your ear and your ankle, with no sagging or bending.

PILLAR BRIDGE FRONT (WIDE FEET)

PROCEDURE: Lift one arm, hold for 2 seconds. Switch arms. Widen your feet, if necessary, to reduce difficulty.

PILLAR BRIDGE FRONT (NARROW FEET)

PROCEDURE: Same exercise as in Level 3. This time, narrow your feet to add to the degree of difficulty.

WWW.COREPERFORMANCE.COM

PILLAR BRIDGE LATERAL

PILLAR BRIDGE LATERAL (KNEELING)

PROCEDURE: Lie on your side with your forearm on the ground and your elbow under your shoulder, with your knees bent to 90 degrees. Push your forearm away from your body, lifting your hips into the air and supporting your weight on your forearm and knees. Hold a static position for the prescribed amount of time. Complete the reps on one side, then switch. **COACHING KEY:** Keep your body in a straight line and keep your stomach tight. If this is too difficult, do individual repetitions – 1 repetition per 2 seconds. **YOU SHOULD FEEL IT:** In your shoulders and trunk.

PILLAR BRIDGE LATERAL

PROCEDURE: Lie on your side with your forearm on the ground under your shoulder, your feet split with the top leg forwards. With your body in a straight line and your elbow under your shoulder, push your hip off the ground, creating a straight line from ankle to shoulder and keeping your head in line with your spine. Hold your position for the prescribed amount of time.

PILLAR BRIDGE LATERAL (STACKED FEET)

PROCEDURE: Instead of splitting your feet, stack them together.

PILLAR BRIDGE LATERAL (JUMPING JACK)

PROCEDURE: From the bridge position, lift your top leg into the air as if you were doing a lateral jumping jack.

GLUTE BRIDGE

GLUTE BRIDGE (MINI BAND)

PROCEDURE: Place a mini band just above your knees. Lying face up on the ground with your arms to your sides, your knees bent and your heels on the ground, lift your hips off the ground until your knees, hips and shoulders are in a straight line. Hold for the prescribed time. If this is too difficult, divide the time into 2- to 3-second intervals, then return to the starting position and repeat until you've completed all of your prescribed time. **COACHING KEY:** Fire (squeeze) your glutes. **YOU SHOULD FEEL IT:** In your glutes, and to a lesser degree in your hamstrings and lower back.

L
E
V
E
L
2

GLUTE BRIDGE (PADDED)

PROCEDURE: Squeeze a rolled-up towel, a doubled-over Thera-Band pad or even a ball between your knees. Lift your hips into the air and then return to the starting position. Repeat for the prescribed number of reps.

L
E
V
E
L
3

GLUTE BRIDGE (MARCHING)

PROCEDURE: Try 'marching' with one leg at a time.

L
E
V
E
L
4

GLUTE BRIDGE (KNEE BENT)

PROCEDURE: Try the Glute Bridge with one leg held to your chest and your weight supported on the other leg. Switch legs.

MINI BAND STANDING

L
E
V
E
L
2

PROCEDURE: Stand with your feet just outside your hips and a mini band above your knees. Move into a partial squat. Keeping your left leg stationary, rotate your right knee in and out for the prescribed number of reps. Then switch legs and repeat. **COACHING KEY:** Keep both feet flat on the ground and your pelvis stable. Don't let the knee of your stationary leg drop inwards. **YOU SHOULD FEEL IT:** In your glutes.

MINI BAND WALKING

L
E
V
E
L
3

PROCEDURE: Move to the right, pushing out with your left leg to create resistance while stepping laterally with your right leg. Bring your left foot back to the starting position and continue until you've completed your reps on that side. Be sure to keep your knees pushed apart throughout the movement. Repeat while moving to the left.

MINI BAND WALKING (ADD RESISTANCE)

L
E
V
E
L
4

PROCEDURE: Increase the resistance by using a band with greater tension.

Ys AND Ts

FLOOR Ys AND Ts

PROCEDURE: Lying face down on the floor with your arms raised slightly above shoulder height, create a Y, with your torso and arms, with your thumbs pointing up. Glide your shoulder blades towards your spine and lift your arms off the ground. Return to the starting position and repeat to complete your reps. For the T, pull your shoulder blades in towards your spine and extend your arms to the sides to create a T. **COACHING KEY:** Keep your stomach tight and your thumbs up. Move from the shoulder blades, not from your arms, extending your shoulders and hands. **YOU SHOULD FEEL IT:** In your shoulders and upper back.

LEVEL 2

PHYSIOBALL Ys AND Ts (ARMS BENT)

PROCEDURE: Perform the same exercise with bent elbows on a physioball, lying face down over the top of the ball so that your back is flat and your chest is off the ball.

LEVEL 3

PHYSIOBALL Ys AND Ts (ARMS EXTENDED)

PROCEDURE: Perform the same exercise as for Level 2, but with your arms extended instead of bent.

LEVEL 4

PHYSIOBALL Ys AND Ts (WITH WEIGHT)

PROCEDURE: Add a light weight – 500 grams to 1.5 kilograms (1 to 3 lbs).

SUMO SQUAT

SUMO SQUAT TO HAMSTRING STRETCH

PROCEDURE: Standing with your feet shoulder width apart, bend at the waist and grab your toes. Drop your hips to the ground, lift your chest up, and then pull your hips forwards until your torso is vertical. Maintaining a flat back, push your hips up and back until you feel a stretch in your hamstrings. Drop your hips back to the ground and repeat until you've completed all your reps. **COACHING KEY:** Keep your chest up, your back flat and your heels on the floor. Keep your elbows inside your knees. For an easier move, place a 1- to 5-centimetre ($^1/_4$- to 2-inch)block under your heels. As your mobility and stability improve, perform the movement with a smaller and smaller heel lift. **YOU SHOULD FEEL:** A stretch in your hamstrings, groin, lower back and quads.

PLATE CRUNCH

PHYSIOBALL PLATE CRUNCH

PROCEDURE: Holding a weight plate, lie on top of the ball and arch your torso backwards. Try to touch your shoulder blades, back and glutes to the ball so that your abdominals are completely stretched. Hold the weight plate behind your head. Roll your hips and chest up at the same time while pulling your belly button in. Crunch from the top of your torso and then lower your hips and chest to the starting position. **COACHING KEY:** Arch your torso completely. **YOU SHOULD FEEL:** A stretch in your abs and core.

PRESS-UP (KNEELING)

L E V E L 2

PROCEDURE: Assume a press-up position with your hands and knees on the ground. Lower your body to the ground, then reverse the movement without touching the ground. Keep your body in a straight line. **COACHING KEY:** Push your sternum as far away from your hands as possible at the end of the movement. **YOU SHOULD FEEL IT:** In your chest, arms and torso.

PRESS-UP

L E V E L 2

PROCEDURE: If you don't need to kneel, assume the normal press-up position.

PRESS-UP (WITH PHYSIOBALL)

L E V E L 3

PROCEDURE: Assume a press-up position, but with your hands on a physioball and your feet on the floor. With your belly button drawn in, lower yourself to the point where your chest barely grazes the ball. Control the ball as you push back up, holding your belly button in and pushing your sternum as far away from the ball as possible. Your shoulder blades should be pushed away from each other in a 'plus' position (as far forwards as possible) at the top of the movement. Keep your fingers pointed down the sides of the ball.

L
E
V
E
L
2

GLUTE BRIDGE (WITH PHYSIOBALL)

PROCEDURE: Lie face up on the ground with your tummy tight and your feet on the ball (or on a bench or a couch). Your legs should be straight, your toes pulled up towards your shins, and your shoulder blades pulled back and down. Contract your glutes to raise your hips until you create a straight line between your ankle and shoulders, so that only your head, shoulders and arms are touching the floor. Hold for 2 to 3 seconds and repeat until you've completed your reps. **COACHING KEY:** Initiate the movement by firing your glutes, and keep them contracted at the top of the movement. If it is too difficult to balance, spread your arms out to the side. Or, to make it more difficult, cross your arms on your chest. **YOU SHOULD FEEL IT:** In your glutes, hamstrings and lower back.

L
E
V
E
L
3

GLUTE BRIDGE (WITH PHYSIOBALL LEG CURL)

PROCEDURE: Contract your glutes to raise your hips, then pull your heels towards your body. Do not let your hips drop as the ball comes towards you. Extend your legs, then repeat the leg curl for the prescribed number of reps without letting your hips touch the ground.

WWW.COREPERFORMANCE.COM

STRENGTH: **CRUNCH**

FLOOR CRUNCH

PROCEDURE: Lie face up with your knees bent, with a small pad or towel under your lower back to help stretch your abs, and your hands behind your head supporting your neck. Lift your chest until your shoulder blades are off the ground, and at the same time rotate your pelvis towards your belly button. Slowly return to the starting position. Repeat until you've completed your reps. **COACHING KEY:** Do not pull on your head with your hands. Feel each segment of your spine flexing as you crunch and as you stretch over the pad. **YOU SHOULD FEEL IT:** In your abdominals.

PHYSIOBALL CRUNCH

PROCEDURE: Lie face up with your body arched over the ball and your hands interlocked, supporting your head. Drape your body over the ball – you should feel a mild stretch in your abs. Curl your trunk and pelvis together while keeping your belly button pulled in. Return to the starting position and repeat until you've completed all your reps.

STRENGTH: **SQUAT**

**L
E
V
E
L
2**

SQUAT (BODY WEIGHT, WITH MINI BAND)

PROCEDURE: Stand with your arms at your sides, your feet shoulder width apart and pointing straight ahead, and a mini band around and above your knees. Maintain perfect posture and initiate movement with your hips. As you reach your arms far forwards, squat your hips back and down until your thighs are parallel to the floor. Return to a standing position by pushing through your hips. Keep your knees out. Repeat until you've completed all your reps. **COACHING KEY:** Keep your knees behind your toes during the movement. Also, keep your knees pushing out against the band so that they do not collapse to the inside during the movement. If you extend your arms in front of you, you can sit back more comfortably. Keep your chest up and your back flat. **YOU SHOULD FEEL IT:** In your glutes, hamstrings and quads.

**L
E
V
E
L
3**

SQUAT (SINGLE LEG, WITH WEIGHTS)

PROCEDURE: Stand on one foot in front of a bench or chair, holding 1- to 2-kilogram (2¹/₂- to 5-lb) weights in each hand. Initiate movement with your hips, squatting back and down on one leg as you reach forwards until your glutes touch the bench. Return to a standing position using only the leg you are balancing on. Repeat for the prescribed number of repetitions, then switch legs. Do not let your knee collapse to the inside.

**L
E
V
E
L
4**

SPLIT SQUAT

PROCEDURE: Hold dumbbells at arm's length at your sides. Place one foot on a box or bench and step out into a lunge with the other. Lower your hips towards the floor by squatting back and down. Without letting your back knee touch the ground, return to the starting position by driving your weight back up with your front leg. Do all the reps with that leg forwards, then switch legs and repeat. **COACHING KEY:** Don't let your front knee slide forwards over your toes; if it does, start over again with your front foot farther forwards. **YOU SHOULD FEEL IT:** In your hips and the fronts of your legs.

SPLIT DUMBBELL CURL

PROCEDURE: In a standing position, hold dumbbells at your side and place one leg on a stable object at about midthigh height. Shift your weight forwards onto your front leg, taking your back leg into a stretch. Now, keeping your elbows still, lift the dumbbells to your shoulders as you rotate your palms to the ceiling. Return to the starting position and repeat until you've completed all your reps. Switch legs midway through the set. **COACHING KEY:** Keep your stomach and the glute muscles of your rear leg tight throughout the movement. Do not allow your back to move. Do not rock forwards or backwards, and don't move your elbows. **YOU SHOULD FEEL IT:** In your biceps, glutes and hip flexors.

SPLIT DUMBBELL CURL TO PRESS

PROCEDURE: After performing a biceps curl, press the weight over your head, finishing with your palms facing forwards. Switch legs midway through the set.

ALTERNATING SPLIT DUMBBELL CURL TO PRESS

PROCEDURE: Stand holding dumbbells at your sides with your front foot resting on a bench or sturdy step at about midthigh height. Push your body weight slightly forwards, with your back glute tight. Perform a biceps curl so that the dumbbells are at your chest. Press your right hand over your head as you lower the left. As you lower your right hand, repeat the motion with your left arm so that the dumbbells pass at your torso. Repeat, switching the foot on the bench halfway through the set. Contract the glute of your back leg to stabilize yourself. Switch legs midway through the set. **COACHING KEY:** Maintain perfect posture, with your belly button pulled in and your shoulder blades pulled back and down. Do not let your back arch when the weight is pressed overhead. **YOU SHOULD FEEL IT:** In your biceps and shoulders, and your pillar.

STANDING LIFT

PROCEDURE: Squat, rotating from right to left while holding a weight plate. Then rotate right, rising back to the starting position, before continuing to rotate and raising the weight plate over your head. **COACHING KEY:** Keep your chest up and your back flat. Lower in the same pattern as you lifted. **YOU SHOULD FEEL IT:** In your hips, torso rotators, upper back, chest and shoulders.

STANDING LIFT (ONE LEG)

PROCEDURE: Stand holding a weight plate or dumbbell in a low position, or holding a rope handle attached to a low pulley cable. Your foot should be perpendicular to the cable if you are using one, your hips should be flexed, and your abdominals should be drawn in. Balance on your inside foot, turn your shoulders and hip towards the leg that's supporting your weight, and keep your chest up and your stomach tight. Squat down so that the weight is outside this leg, then fire from your glutes and torso. Pull the weight or handles towards your chest while extending your supporting leg. Turn your trunk away from your supporting leg as your hands push up and away. Return to the starting position and repeat to complete your reps, then switch legs. **COACHING KEY:** Keep your chest up and your back flat. Your torso will rotate from start to finish. This exercise combines the movements of balance squatting, rotating, the upright row and the incline press. Lower in the same pattern as you lifted. **YOU SHOULD FEEL IT:** In your hips, torso rotators, upper back, chest and shoulders.

ALTERNATING DUMBBELL BENCH PRESS

PROCEDURE: Lie face up on a bench, holding dumbbells at the outside edges of your shoulders, your palms facing your thighs. Lift the dumbbells straight up over your chest. Keeping one arm straight, lower the other dumbbell, touch the outside of your shoulder, then push it back up. Switch arms and continue to alternate arms for the prescribed number of reps. **COACHING KEY:** Keep your non-working arm straight. Keep your feet on the floor and your hips and shoulders on the bench at all times. Pull your stomach in to stabilize your core. **YOU SHOULD FEEL IT:** In your chest, shoulders and triceps.

ROMANIAN DEADLIFT (TWO ARMS, ONE LEG)

PROCEDURE: Stand on one foot while holding a dumbbell in each hand, using an overhand grip. 'Hinge' over at the waist, lowering the dumbbells as your nonsupporting leg lifts behind you. Return to the standing position by contracting your hamstrings and glutes. Repeat for the prescribed number of repetitions, then switch legs. **COACHING KEY:** Do not let your back arch. Your torso and leg should move as one unit. Fire the glute of your extended leg to keep it straight. Keep your shoulder blades back and down throughout the movement, and keep the dumbbells close to your shin. **YOU SHOULD FEEL IT:** In your glutes, hamstrings and back.

ONE-ARM, ONE-LEG DUMBBELL ROW

PROCEDURE: Stand on your right leg, hinged over at the waist, holding a dumbbell with your right hand and holding on to a stable, waist-high surface with your left hand. Lift your left leg to form a *T* with your body. Slide your right shoulder blade towards your spine and then lift the weight to your body by driving your elbow to the ceiling. Return to the starting position and repeat for the prescribed number of repetitions. Then switch sides. **COACHING KEY:** Move with your shoulder, not your arm, to initiate the row. Keep your back level – your shoulders should stay parallel to the floor – and fire the glute of your extended leg to keep it parallel to the floor. Extend the leg opposite the hand doing the lifting. **YOU SHOULD FEEL IT:** In your back, lats and shoulders.

ACKNOWLEDGMENTS

Writing a book, like the Game of Life, is a team effort. This book would not have been completed were it not for a talented team of people playing their positions exceptionally well.

That team could fill the largest locker room, and space prohibits me from thanking everyone by name. I must, however, single out the staff, athletes and extended family of Athletes' Performance for their input and inspiration. Special thanks go to Amanda Carlson, Craig Friedman and Dan Burns for helping to shape the message of this programme. I am also grateful for the insights from our friends at Tignum (*www.tignum.com*), namely Hans-Jürgen Rippel and Scott Peltin. Debbie Martell, the wonderful performance chef at Athletes' Performance, provided a huge assist with the recipes in this book. As always, I owe a huge debt of gratitude to my co-conspirators David Black and Pete Williams, along with Rodale's team of Jeremy Katz, Pete Fornatale, Susan Eugster, Karen Neely, Susannah Hogendorn and Jennifer Giandomenico for helping me to fulfil the goal of sharing the Core message with others. Last of all to my beautiful wife, Amy; our family; and our Athletes' Performance team.

INDEX

Boldface page references indicate photographs and illustrations.

Underscored references indicate boxed text.

ABOUT THE AUTHORS

Mark Verstegen is recognized as one of the world's most innovative sports performance experts. As the owner of Athletes' Performance – cutting-edge training centres in Tempe, Arizona, and Carson, California – he directs teams of performance specialists and nutritionists to train some of the most recognized names in sport.

By teaching an integrated lifestyle and training programme that blends strength, speed, flexibility, joint and 'core' stability and mental toughness, Verstegen helps athletes become not only faster and stronger but also more powerful, flexible and resistant to injury and long-term back, hip and other joint problems.

Because of his innovative techniques and up-to-date knowledge of sporting performance,

Verstegen is a sought-after consultant. He serves as director of performance for the NFL Players Association, is an advisor to Adidas, EAS, Amino Vital and other leading performance-oriented companies, and serves as a consultant to numerous athletic governing bodies.

A dynamic speaker, Verstegen travels the world to address groups such as the American College of Sports Medicine, the National Strength and Conditioning Association and many corporate audiences.

Verstegen and his training methods have been profiled by dozens of national media outlets. He's a contributing columnist to *Men's Health*® magazine and the executive producer of fitness programmes for Sportskool, America's first video-on-demand cable network dedicated to expert sport and fitness instruction. His first book, *Core Performance: The Revolutionary Workout Programme to Transform Your Body and Your Life,* was published by Rodale in 2004 and soared to as high as No. 24 on the Amazon.com bestseller list.

Verstegen began his coaching career at his alma mater, Washington State University, following a career-ending football injury. He served as assistant director of player development at Georgia Tech and in 1994 created the International Performance Institute on the campus of the IMG Sports Academy in Bradenton, Florida. In 1999, he moved to Phoenix to build Athletes' Performance, which quickly became the industry leader for training world-class athletes.

Verstegen and his wife, Amy, live in Scottsdale, Arizona.

Pete Williams is a veteran journalist who has written about sport, business and fitness for numerous publications, including *USA Today,* the *Washington Post,* and Street & Smith's *SportsBusiness Journal.* He is the author of two books on the sports memorabilia business – *Card Sharks* and *Sports Memorabilia for Dummies* – and is co-author of two previous Rodale books: *Core Performance* (with Mark Verstegen) and *Fun Is Good* (with Mike Veeck). A graduate of the University of Virginia, he lives in Florida with his wife, Suzy, and sons, Luke and Lance.

For more information on Mark Verstegen's Core training programmes, including interactive workouts and nutritional plans, please visit *www.coreperformance.com.* The site also offers sport-specific, DVD programmes for tennis, golf, football and other sports, along with Core training equipment and information on how to attend seminars and personalized training weeks at Athletes' Performance in Tempe, Arizona, and Carson, California.

For more information on Pete Williams, please visit *www.petewilliams.net.*